LAUGH WHILE YOU LEARN

Go To
DavidMeinz.com
to watch David's Free Videos

Although the author and publisher have exhaustively researched all sources to ensure the accuracy and completeness of the information contained in this book, we assume no responsibility for errors, inaccuracies, omissions or any inconsistency herein. This publication is not designed to take the place of medical advice by a competent professional. Consult your physician and registered dietitian before adopting any health suggestions in this book. The ideas, procedures, and suggestions in this book are intended to supplement, not replace, the medical advice of a trained professional. Any slights of people or organizations are unintentional. The author and publisher disclaim any liability arising directly or indirectly from the use of this book.

Copyright © MMXV by David L. Meinz

All rights reserved. No portion of this book may be reproduced or transmitted in any form or by any means, electronic or mechanical, including photocopying, recording, or by an information storage and retrieval system—except by a reviewer who may quote brief passages in a review to be printed in a magazine or newspaper—without the written permission of the author. For information, please contact Gilbert Press, P.O. Box 772525, Orlando, FL 32877

Published in Orlando, Florida, by Gilbert Press

1st Edition
First printing, MMXV
ISBN 978-0-9644253-1-6

TEN BONUS YEARS

How You Can Add 10 HEALTHY YEARS To Your Life

David L. Meinz
MS, RDN, FAND, CSP

"Ten Bonus Years" is available for
quantity purchases at a significant discount.
Customized print runs for businesses
and organizations are also available.
For information, contact:
Gilbert Press, P.O. Box 772525, Orlando, FL 32877
1-800-488-2857

TABLE OF CONTENTS

INTRODUCTION 1

PART 1 – THE LONGEVITY RECIPE..........7

A LONG & HEALTHY LIFE 9

1. Have A Reason To Get Up In The Morning............................ 10
2. Make Family And Friends A High Priority 15
3. Put More Physical Activity Into Your Lifestyle 22
4. Maintain A Healthy Weight................... 30
5. Start Eating More Plant-Based Foods........ 45
6. Eat More Nuts!............................. 53
7. Learn To Handle Stress 69
8. Realize That There Is A Spiritual Dimension To Life 78
9. Stop Blaming Your Parents.................. 80
10. Beat The Two Big Killers 88

PART 2 – CHAMPIONS OF LONGEVITY ... 93

LONG-LIVED AMERICANS 95

TABLE OF CONTENTS CON'T

PART 3 – BEAT HEART DISEASE 103

DON'T TRUST YOUR CHOLESTEROL NUMBER 105

    Live The Good Life........................... 108

    Take A Shot 110

    Act Like A Baby 111

    Suck It In 113

    Don't Resist................................. 115

    You're Just Getting Started................... 118

PART 4– PREVENT CANCER 121

OVER A HALF MILLION A YEAR 123

    2015 Estimated US Female/Male
       Cancer Deaths (table)..................... 129

    Trends In US Female Cancer Deaths
       1930-2011 (table) 130

    Trends In US Male Cancer Deaths
       1930-2011 (table) 131

PART 5 – EAT LIKE AN ITALIAN 133

LET'S MEET IN THE MIDDLE 135

It's Good And Good For You.................... 137
Here's What You Should Eat.................. 141
Not Popeye's Girlfriend 143
I'll Drink To That?............................ 148
That Was Then, This Is Now.................. 150
Eating Like Them, Over Here................. 154
The Big Picture.............................. 159

CONCLUSION 161

TEN BONUS YEARS

INTRODUCTION

IMAGINE sometime in the future, you're in the hospital and your doctor says that you only have 24 hours left to live. This is it. You've come to the end of your journey. The moment we all know will someday come, has now come for you. Soon your family is gathered around you, solemn, tearful, and preparing to say goodbye.

Now what if I showed up at your bedside and told you I could give you 10 more years, 10 bonus healthy years. 10 more vibrant years, full of life! Would you listen to what I had to say? You would.

Well, it won't work if you wait till you're on your deathbed. But recent research shows that if you'll take several simple steps now you can add 10 bonus years to your life.

What would ten extra healthy years mean to you?

It might mean getting to see your grandchildren grow up. It might mean seeing them get married. It might mean getting to know your great-grandchildren. It might mean dramatically decreasing your chances of having a heart attack, stroke, or cancer. It might mean not leaving your spouse as a widow or widower. And it might mean having a mind and body that still works great as you get older. It might mean ten healthy extra years to really enjoy life. You have the potential for all of that.

> **THE LONGEST LIVING PERSON IN MODERN TIMES WAS A FRENCH WOMAN NAMED JEANNE CALMENT. SHE CELEBRATED 122 BIRTHDAYS!**

Her mind was sharp and her body worked pretty well too. As a matter of fact, she rode her bicycle everyday until she was 110! She attended opera, played tennis, enjoyed swimming and hunting, and even roller-skating.

Let's be honest, you might not initially be interested in living 10 extra years. A lot of people think living older means living in a nursing home. But that's all changing. The number of older Americans with chronic disability is actually going down. And that's in spite of the fact that Americans are living longer than ever. There's even been a 22 percent decrease in nursing home use. Only about 5 percent of people over age 65 actually live in nursing homes. Not only have there been advancements in medical care, but a lot of older people are taking better care of themselves. More than eight out of 10 people over the age of 65 can take care of themselves in daily living without any outside help. Remember, John Glenn went back to space when he was 77! It pays to take care of yourself. A study of 1700 people reported in the *New England Journal of Medicine* found that people with healthier habits had only half as much disability during the two years before their deaths as those with the poorest health habits. People in their 80's today are by far healthier than people in their 80's a generation or two ago. Most people today in their 80's don't report any serious disabilities.

122 year-old Jeanne Calment didn't act like an old person. How about you? Are you acting your age? Hopefully not. It's important to remember that while you have to get older, you don't necessarily need to get old.

Your second fifty years may be better than the

first fifty years. Since your odds of living healthier as you get older are better than you may have originally thought, I hope you'll take the steps necessary to have both quality and quantity of life. Mickey Mantle once said "If I knew I was going to live this long, I would've taken better care of myself." More than half of today's 74 million baby boomers will live past age 85, but they will suffer with chronic diseases unless they change their ways. You don't have to be one of them.

You and I probably won't make it to 122. But we definitely can live ten healthy years longer than most other people.

A poll conducted by ABC News and *USA Today* asked Americans how long they would like to live. The average responder said 87 years, which is nine years longer than the current national average. Would you take an extra year to make it an even 10? Are you interested? I hope you are. Now is the time when you can add those ten extra healthy years to your life. Let's get started!

INTRODUCTION

PART 1: THE LONGEVITY RECIPE

1
THE LONGEVITY RECIPE

A LONG & HEALTHY LIFE

There are more healthy long-lived people on the Japanese island of Okinawa than any other place in the world. Per square mile, there are also more healthy 100-year-olds than any other place on the planet. Based on what's been learned from them and other long-lived population groups around the world, longevity researchers have discovered characteristics that seem to be universally associated with longevity. While, of course, there's no absolute guarantee that practicing these will add years to your life, you will definitely be increasing your odds that your life will be longer and healthier.

By the way, remember that whenever you try to make behavior changes, you want to make those changes convenient to your lifestyle. Research shows that if you stick with a new habit for five weeks it's more likely to become part of your routine. Other research indicates twelve weeks. So somewhere between five and twelve weeks of dedication is what's required for a new practice to become a habit. Start with those new behaviors that are easier to accomplish and then build on success. Here's what we've learned from people around the world who live long and healthy lives.

1. HAVE A REASON TO GET UP IN THE MORNING

Do something that you feel is important, worthwhile, or interesting. The very old healthy people from Okinawa, Japan call it "ikigai." Long-lived healthy people often have a strong sense of purpose. They feel needed and that they're making a contribution. That purpose can be something that's important just to you; you don't have to change the world. If working in your garden gets you excited, that's all it takes. A recent eleven-year study funded by the National Institutes of Health found that those individuals that had a clear goal in life did, in fact, live longer and were mentally sharper than those who did not.

The New York City health department found that 46 percent more people died during the first week of the year 2000 than the last week of the year 1999. It's commonly believed by researchers now that many people had a personal goal to make it to the 21st century. That desire may have actually helped them stay alive. You probably know of stories of older or sick people who stayed around until after a birthday or a wedding or some other important holiday was completed. Your mind can affect your health.

Another study that looked at over 12,000 middle-aged Hungarians discovered that those who felt that their lives had a purpose had much lower rates of heart disease and cancer than those that didn't feel that way. Professor Harold Koenig, M.D. of Duke University discovered that people who have a feeling of being part of a larger plan in life and are guided by their spiritual values have a stronger immune system, a lower risk of heart attack and cancer, and lower blood pressure. They also heal faster, and they live longer, too.

For many people, we get our purpose from our job or career. In fact, a European study that looked at over 16,000 people for twelve years found a 51 percent higher rate of dying in those who retire early than in those who kept on working. Now it's true, some people who retire early may do so because of poor health. So it may be the poor health of those people, not the fact that they retired early, that contributed to their earlier death. Nevertheless, a lot of research does indicate that staying engaged in life is good for you. By the way, you've probably heard that people who work all the time are at higher risk for health problems. Interestingly, there is no evidence that workaholics are at a higher health risk if they really enjoy what they're doing. Engagement seems to make the difference.

So even if you don't need to work for a living anymore, you may still benefit by finding something to do. Once you officially "retire" you may have the time to really pursue your passion. Take time to figure out what that is. What's really important to you in life? Ask yourself who the people are in life that you really admire. It may be what you really admire about them is what they do. Can you do something similar? If money wasn't a problem or an issue, what would you really *like* to do?

Keep in mind today that the average 60-year-old will live to be about 83. If you're younger than

PART 1: THE LONGEVITY RECIPE

60, the average expected lifespan is even more than that. Lots of us will live into our 90's. That means a whole bunch of us are going to be "officially retired" for almost a third of our lives. Many people put a lot of planning into the finances of retirement. They make sure there's going to be enough money. But even when they're successful doing that, the average person who retires starts to get bored after about four to six months. Then they're always looking for something to do. You don't want the last third of your life spent watching *M*A*S*H* reruns or *Wheel of Fortune* every day.

GIVING BACK CAN BE GOOD FOR YOUR HEALTH, TOO. RESEARCHERS AT PURDUE UNIVERSITY FOUND THAT DEPRESSED OLDER PEOPLE IMPROVED THEIR MOODS WHEN THEY VOLUNTEERED.

If you decide to volunteer, make sure it's for something that you think is important. Staying interested and intellectually engaged keeps you sharp and slows down mental decline. For your health's sake, and so you live long enough to enjoy the money you worked so hard for, you may want to spend some time planning exactly what it is you want to do for that last third of your life.

For some great ideas on making sure your money and your health last as long as you do—be sure to get a copy of my book *Wealthy, Healthy & Wise*. You can get it at www.DavidMeinz.com.

So think about it, why do you get up in the morning? Right now it may be to pay off your mortgage. Hopefully, someday that will be paid. Why don't you take some time and figure out what's really important in your life. Write down the mission statement for *you*. Your personal purpose can come from your faith or your hobby or your job or whatever else you're passionate about. And consider acquiring a new skill. Learning a new language or how to play a musical instrument not only gives you a goal but also seems to keep your brain sharper for a longer period. It's "exercising your brain." Decide to work toward your personal mission in life a little every day. It'll probably make that life longer and healthier, too.

2. MAKE FAMILY AND FRIENDS A HIGH PRIORITY

Almost all long-lived healthier older folks have been married and had children. Their lives tend to revolve around a large family and many live with their extended multi-generational families. They get better care and they both receive and give love. We know that children do better growing up if they live in households with grandparents present. Except in the United States, it's usually considered dishonorable to send an elderly relative to a nursing home. In Okinawa, where they participate in religion that includes ancestor worship, many gravesites actually have picnic tables where family members can come by and celebrate meals with deceased relatives!

Older people that live with their extended families are healthier; they eat better, they have less stress and disease, and they're less likely to be involved in serious accidents. They also tend to stay more mentally sharp. The long-lived Okinawans often get together with a large number of relatives on a regular basis. The occasion is usually a celebration of the health and good fortune of the oldest living member of the family. Sometimes we Americans do the same thing at a family reunion. We probably need to do it more often.

Staying socially connected with friends is good for your longevity, too. It tends to improve your outlook, builds self-confidence, and helps you get through stressful times.

> **SOME STUDIES SHOW THAT AT ANY GIVEN AGE, THOSE WITH FEW FRIENDSHIPS OR RELATIONSHIPS HAVE TWICE THE RISK OF DYING.**

Research shows that the average American only has two close personal friends that they can really count on. That can contribute to an increasing sense of stress and isolation.

My mom goes to a "donut group" once a week. She meets with some of her senior citizen friends and they each have one or two donuts. The donuts are really just an excuse to get together and visit. Even though she's eating high sugar and high fat, the benefit she gets from socializing with a group of friends probably does her more good than the donuts do her damage. She's recently been complaining that a lot in her group, which originally had about twenty members, have died. They're now down to about six. I suggested to her that it may have something to do with all the donuts they eat. She didn't think that was it.

Those relationships you have with the people you see every day seem to have the greatest impact on your health. The research is clear that committed marriage that includes love and mutual respect is good for your health as well. Married people live longer than the single, the divorced, or those that are widowed. The benefit doesn't come just from the legal binding marriage certificate, of course, but in the quality of the relationship. One of the reasons that the surviving spouse often dies shortly after the first spouse dies is probably related to the health benefit we get from that close social relationship.

But marriage can also harm your health if it's not a good one. Scientists at Ohio State University Medical School observed 90 married couples and found that those who had the most hostility and negativity during their discussions showed a dramatic decrease in immune function over the next 24 hours. They also found that women who had been separated or divorced had a decrease in immune function as well.

Fortunately, they also found the opposite. Those that have good communication skills and relationships seem to benefit with a boost to the immune system. Interestingly, marriage seems to be more helpful to men than women. In fact, divorced men have higher death rates than widowed men or men that were never married. Women, on the other hand, seem to get more health protection from relationships with friends and relatives. Those tend to often be with other women.

Positive human contact and support is absolutely essential for a healthy long life. Humans need other humans. It's just that simple. People who care about you may encourage you to practice better health habits, too.

Dr. James House, of the University of Michigan says that the research suggests that a lack of social relationships constitutes a major risk factor for health. He says the effect is similar to other risk factors such as cigarette smoking, high blood pressure, obesity, blood lipid levels, and physical inactivity. He says our current understanding of the impact of social relationships on health and longevity is about where we were in our understanding of tobacco's impact on health back in 1964. That's saying a lot.

So, just what is social support? In general, it's a

person's belief that he or she is loved, esteemed, cared for, and part of a mutual caring network.

Regardless of your age, the risk of death is 2-4 times higher in those that are socially isolated than in those who are socially connected to other people. Those people that have cardiovascular disease but also have a good network of family and friends are more likely to recover from a heart attack, stroke or heart surgery.

> **BEING SOCIALLY ISOLATED IS ASSOCIATED WITH A HIGHER RISK OF ARTHRITIS, HEART DISEASE, DEPRESSION, ALCOHOLISM, SUICIDE, AND OTHER PHYSICAL AND EMOTIONAL PROBLEMS.**

For people in their 60's, 70's, and 80's research has shown that having family and friends in your life helps you maintain both your physical and mental health. You're more likely to avoid depression and disability, too.

As you'll soon learn, people who attend church regularly live longer. A personal faith seems to help people deal with the challenges of life. Most religions are based on a hope for a better future.

People who go to church tend to have a greater support group and tend to have lower stress levels, a more positive outlook, and are generally more at peace with the world.

> **RESEARCHERS AT DUKE UNIVERSITY FOUND THAT PEOPLE WHO ATTENDED RELIGIOUS SERVICES AT LEAST ONCE A WEEK HAD HEALTHIER IMMUNE SYSTEMS.**

We've seen the importance of relationships lived out in the small town of Roseto, Pennsylvania. Just north of Philadelphia, this town is made up of the descendents of those who immigrated from southern Italy back in the 1880's. Over the years they've maintained close family ties, church membership, multi-generation households, and a strong cultural identity.

Researchers discovered that even though the residents of Roseto historically had diets very high in fat, their death rates from heart disease were low. Even when other traditional health factors were accounted for, there was no other explanation of the resident's protection except for their strong social ties. Interestingly, in more recent years the residents of Roseto have been adopting healthier lower fat diets but they have also become more mobile like the rest of America. There are less multi-generational families in town and the residents are starting to look like the rest of homogenized America. In spite of healthier habits, as their social ties have decreased, their heart disease rates have started to go up.

If you're like a lot of Americans, working on friendships may seem like a relatively low priority; especially if you're a male. We're just not into all that. And besides, we're busy. But the research is clear that quality relationships in your life with both family and friends can help you live both a longer life and a healthier life.

Dedicate some time to maintaining and creating good relationships. Look for classes to go to or organizations that share a passion that you do. Take a cooking class. Volunteer. You'll be healthier because of it. When retirement time comes, those communities that are designed for those 55 years and over are a great idea, too. You'll have a built-in extended support group and lots of activities. There's no reason to feel alone.

3. PUT MORE PHYSICAL ACTIVITY INTO YOUR LIFESTYLE

If you've been looking for that elusive fountain of youth it may be exercise. It reduces your chances of obesity, heart disease, stroke, certain cancers, and osteoporosis. What's more, exercise improves your mood and mental outlook so much that many physicians recommend it as a treatment for depression. One study found that being inactive gives you the same risk for heart disease as if you smoked one pack of cigarettes a day.

Most long-lived healthy people have regular low intensity physical activity as part of their routine. You need a combination of aerobic, muscle strengthening activities, and balancing. Keeping in mind that falling is a common reason for injuries and deaths among senior citizens in the United States, yoga is a great exercise that can help with that balance.

Walking is one of the best exercises you can do;

PART 1: THE LONGEVITY RECIPE 23

it doesn't cost anything, and it's available any time you want to do it. But the most important thing is to find some activity that you enjoy. For me personally, I watch movies while I'm on my exercise bike. I don't like riding the exercise bike, but I do like watching movies. I don't concentrate on exercising, I concentrate on the movie. The time goes by much faster that way.

For a long time it was believed that as a person got older it was inevitable that they would lose muscle, bone, and strength and that those changes were irreversible. Now it's true that your muscles will usually get smaller and weaker as you get older. Sedentary people lose approximately 40 percent of their muscle mass and 30 percent of their strength between the ages of 20 and 70. Unless, that is, you do strength training exercises. If you don't build muscle, you will lose muscle. Starting at about age 20, you begin to slowly lose muscle mass. That contributes to a lower metabolic rate and an increase in body fat. Even aerobic exercise does not prevent muscle mass loss; it takes resistive exercise and strength training. Men and women who do strength training as they get older are much less likely to fall and break a bone due to poor balance, poor gait, or loss of muscle strength.

The idea that we all inevitably go down hill as we get older all changed in the 1990's when researchers found that, after only eight weeks of three exercise sessions a week, frail nursing home residents between the ages of 86 and 96 actually increased their muscular strength by 175 percent. They improved their walking speed and balance as well. Some of them were even able to throw away their canes! What's interesting is that these improvements in strength did not come from bigger muscles, but by simply allowing their bodies to more effectively use the muscles they already had. The strength of their leg muscles more than doubled, the seniors became more mobile, and they increased their activity level as well. In addition, those who lifted weights expended 15 percent more calories which helped them with weight loss. Also important, their bodies held on to 15 percent more of the protein they ate. Since lifting weights causes muscles to get bigger, the body better utilizes the protein that is consumed. A study at Tufts University looked at 40 healthy, but sedentary, post-menopausal women. They participated just twice a week, in 40-minute weightlifting sessions. After one year, the women's bodies were 15 to 20 years more youthful. They actually gained bone density at an age when women typically lose bone.

PART 1: THE LONGEVITY RECIPE

In another study, 70-year-old men who had done strength training since middle age were just as strong, on average, as 28-year-olds who did not exercise. 70-year-olds just as strong as 28-year-olds. That's amazing!

A 1998 study reported in the *New England Journal of Medicine* looked at 700 elderly men.

> **THOSE WHO WALKED MORE THAN TWO MILES A DAY HAD HALF THE DEATH RATE OVER 12 YEARS AS THOSE WHO WALKED LESS THAN ONE MILE.**

This especially lowered cancer risk. Exercise may decrease cancer risk by improving immune function and hormone levels. Two or three miles a day at a moderate rate is doable for most seniors. Remember, if you walk with a friend you're not only getting exercise but you're also getting social interaction. That's a win-win situation for everyone.

A study reported in the *Journal of the American Medical Association* found that women who exercise at least four hours a week had a 37 percent lower risk of breast cancer than sedentary women. One guess is that moderate exercise may lower estrogen and progestin levels, thereby inhibiting malignant changes in the breast. Since fat tissue is a source of estrogen, and since exercise reduces body fat, exercise may also be working that way as well.

Exercise can reduce blood pressure and inflammation, improve cholesterol levels, cut the risk of life-threatening diseases, and normalize insulin levels.

Activity can help keep your mind sharp as you get older, too. Part of the problem of dementia in the elderly is a decrease in blood flow to the brain. Of course, regular exercise can improve this. If exercise was a pill, everyone would take it.

IN FACT, THE DATA IS STRONGER FOR THE IMPACT OF EXERCISE ON YOUR BRAIN THAN THE ASSOCIATION BETWEEN NUTRITION AND BRAIN HEALTH.

A study that looked at 2000 people over 25 years found that those that had been more fit as young adults scored better on mental tests when they reached middle age. Fortunately, the results also showed that those that improved their fitness as they got older also scored well.

Much of what many people believed to be old age

is not age related at all. The average decline in functional ability so many people experience with age is the result of a lack of physical activity and poor dietary habits over a lifetime. What we're learning now is that a lot of that damage can be reversed. The body has an amazing ability to bounce back. That means that it's never too late to start! There is enormous benefit from exercising just by going from the least active category to the next level up. Just start doing something. Remember, older people who are more physically fit not only live longer, but more importantly, they live healthier, better quality lives.

Aim for at least 30 minutes of moderate exercise five days a week; about 150 minutes total per week. A brisk walk would be considered a moderate intensity activity. For more intense exercise, like a treadmill, jogging, or a stationary bike, 75 minutes a week is a good minimum. That's per week, not per day. More is certainly OK, but most Americans don't even get the suggested minimums. A good target is to try for about 2000 exercise calories burned per week. One study at Stanford University found that those who exercised at that level by walking, climbing stairs, and playing sports decreased their death rate by 28 percent. Remember activity includes aerobic exercise, strength training, and flexibility. Aerobic exercise should be intense enough to make you break a sweat and breathe hard. Resistance strength training, like lifting weights or using a weight machine, is recommended at three times a week. Do 1-3 sets of 8-12 repetitions for each muscle group. By the way, strength training will not hurt most people with arthritis because it does not cause the bones to rub against each other like aerobics does. For stretching and flexibility, stretch the major muscle groups to the point of mild discomfort but not to where you feel pain. Overstretch for approximately 20 seconds and do not bounce during a stretch. Several minutes of stretching 3-5 days a week is a good idea.

One of the most significant benefits of regular exercise is that it decreases what is called "visceral" fat. This is the fat that collects in your midsection around your vital organs. It's not the same as subcutaneous fat that collects under the skin and around the hips and thighs. You may not like the looks of subcutaneous fat, but it's not near as dangerous as the kind of fat you don't see in your insides. That's why today we tell people to measure their waist size. It's that dangerous visceral fat that tends to make your mid-section bigger. Women should not go above 35 inches, and men should not go above 40 inches. It's at that point that your health risks start to go up dramatically. The research indicates you need a 45-minute brisk walk five days a week, or its equivalent in other exercise, to see a decrease in this middle or visceral fat.

And here's something else that's important. Just because you're thin does not mean you're necessarily fit.

> **RESEARCH IS CLEAR THAT BEING FIT EVEN IF YOU ARE MODERATELY OVERWEIGHT IS STILL BETTER THAN BEING SKINNY AND UNFIT.**

So even if you can't lose all the weight you want to by exercise, you are getting fit along the way. That fitness, in and of itself, is protective of your health.

By the way, statistically speaking, people who do serious exercise only gain a year or two of extra life. That doesn't sound like much. But keep in mind that's an average. On an individual basis, and from all the health benefits that come from exercise, the increase in lifespan could potentially be a decade or more. And, again, those years are likely to be healthier years, too. And that makes it worth putting exercise into your life.

4. MAINTAIN A HEALTHY WEIGHT

Taking body fat off your body is incredibly easy to understand. And for most people it's incredibly hard to do. What's even harder to do is to keep the weight off, once it's off. In the vast majority of cases, long-term weight control really is about how many calories you take in versus how many calories you burn off. The good news is that if you understand some basics it's easier to decrease the amount of calories you eat than it is to burn calories off once you've eaten them. For example, many people with a weight problem are not overeating quantities of food. What they are doing is eating foods that have high caloric density. That is to say, they have a lot of calories in a small amount of food. The culprit in jamming a lot of calories into food is usually either sugar or fat, or both. Consider that 1 cup of pasta, like fettuccini, has 220 calories. But 1 cup of Alfredo sauce has a whopping 996 calories! And 100 grams of fat! It's the fat in the sauce that's the real source of calories. And what gets the blame for being

PART 1: THE LONGEVITY RECIPE 31

fattening? The pasta. Not guilty! An average size baked potato has 194 calories, but put some sour cream and butter on top and you double the calories! Once again, the fat, not the potato is the problem. When you reduce the amount of fat in a food, you can still get the same amount of food with a lot less calories. A cup of whole milk has 170 calories but the same cup of 1 percent milk only has 100 calories. And consider that one apple has about 53 calories. But a slice of apple pie has 285 calories. Basically the same food, but the pie has lots of sugar and fat added.

The point is not to avoid apple pie, but to realize that both will fill you up, but with significant differences to your waistline. Whole-grain, whole foods with fiber tend to have more volume to them than their white flour, processed counterparts. Foods in the form closer to the way they grow fill you up quicker without giving you a lot of calories. Brown rice fills you up better than white rice. Whole wheat bread fills you up better than white bread.

By the way, despite the common notion that they cause weight gain, there is nothing uniquely fattening about breads, cereals, rice, and potatoes. Most of the world eats more carbohydrates than Americans, yet Americans are fatter than anybody else on earth. The average citizen of China has traditionally had a rice-based diet; lots of carbohydrate. But there has never been an obesity problem in China, that is, until recently when they started eating more Western type foods. The average Italian eats four times more bread than the average American but you still don't see the obesity levels in Europe as you do in the US. True, there are some fat people over there, but those are the American tourists!

You'll also do yourself a favor if you'll slow down a little when you eat. It takes about twenty minutes for your brain to realize that your stomach is full. So if you stop eating when you're about 80 percent full you give your brain a chance to catch up with the signals being sent by your stomach. If you do that you'll find that the amount of food you've already eaten is plenty. If you eat until your full you've gone too far. You really need to be aware of what's going on while you're eating. Personally, I know that there are times when I'm eating that I've had enough, but there's still food on my plate. Since I was raised to not waste food, I keep on eating till my plate is clean.

You can use smaller plates and smaller glasses, too. I know it sounds silly, but research has shown that if you use smaller plates, bowls, and glasses you can decrease your intake by about 30 percent.

And without being hungry. Americans tend to fill up their plates, and then clean up their plates. Use smaller plates and don't worry, you can go back for seconds if you're still hungry.

If you'll slow down when you eat, and pay attention to your body, instead of the TV or your email, you may find you're quite satisfied with a smaller amount of food and calories. That's a lot easier than trying to burn the calories off. Of course, physical activity IS essential for long-term weight control. But the purpose of exercise is not just to burn calories, but to make whole-body changes in your metabolism that will allow weight loss.

> **THE IMPORTANT LESSON IS THAT MOST AMERICANS STOP EATING WHEN THEIR STOMACHS FEEL FULL, MOST NORMAL WEIGHT PEOPLE STOP EATING WHEN THEY'RE NO LONGER HUNGRY.**

That's a big difference. You combine that way of eating with eating less high sugar and fat foods, and you've got the formula for long-term weight control success.

Among researchers, there is an ongoing debate on whether or not being a little overweight is dangerous for your longevity. A lot of research over the years has said that the best weight for longevity is right at ideal body weight or even a few pounds under. But the most recent research would suggest that even if you are obese with a BMI between 30 or 40, even that probably does not decrease your longevity. That's right, does not decrease your longevity. (To calculate your BMI, multiply your weight by 700. Then divide that by your height in inches. Then divide that by your height in inches again. That number is your BMI.) That does not, however, mean you're healthy.

> **IT'S CLEAR THAT PEOPLE WHO ARE OVERWEIGHT ARE MORE LIKELY TO HAVE HIGH BLOOD PRESSURE, HIGH CHOLESTEROL, DIABETES, ARTHRITIS, HEART DISEASE, CANCER, AND A HOST OF OTHER PROBLEMS.**

Ironically, we have enough drugs today to keep obese unhealthy people alive. But living on drugs is clearly not the way to live if you don't have to. Remember, most people agree that quality of life is even more important than actual quantity of life. What the research does show, however, is that if you have a BMI of 40 or greater, what we call extreme obesity, you definitely do decrease your lifespan.

For example, an extremely obese 40-year-old man can expect to live nine years less than someone the same age who is normal weight. Nine years. By the way, if you're extremely obese the last thing you want to do is smoke. If you do smoke, and you're extremely obese, the research indicates that it's going to cut 21 years off your life expectancy. Yes, 21 years. It's not cheap being overweight either. An obese individual spends about $1400 more per year in medical bills compared to the average healthy person. And even though you may not necessarily die quicker, being overweight may make you get older quicker. Researchers at the University of Medicine and Dentistry of New Jersey measured the telomere length between obese and lean women. Telomeres are the end like caps on chromosomes that keep them from fraying and becoming unstable and more likely to mutate. The shorter telomeres become, the more you age. Everything else being equal, they found the obese women had shorter telomeres. In other words, obesity was making the women age quicker. Once again, we're talking quality of life.

So the bottom line is that if you're willing to take a lot of medicines over most of your life and put up with their side effects and expense, and the side effects of being overweight, then being overweight, and maybe even moderately obese, may not necessarily take away years from your lifespan. It most likely, however, will take away from the enjoyment and quality of life you have from those years. Medical science is good enough now to keep you medicated to keep you going. But it appears that only you can determine the quality of years that you'll have. Don't get confused by all these viewpoints. Aim for your ideal body weight. If you can't do that, the research indicates that if you lose as little as 10 percent of your current body weight you still can expect health improvement. Just 10 percent of your current weight. Do something. Don't be complacent just because most of the people you know are also overweight. When it comes to your health, you don't want to look like the average American.

In spite of all the problems that obesity causes in America today, we have an even greater problem in this country with obesity in children. Obesity rates are increasing faster in children than any other age group. An adult who gains weight from middle age on could certainly expect health problems as a result later in life. However, when obesity starts in childhood, those children are exposed to the impact of that obesity over an entire lifetime. As a result, we're already seeing teenagers with diabetes and young people with heart attacks in their 30's. And that, unfortunately, appears to just be the tip of the iceberg. Keep in mind, that most of the obese adults today were at least normal weight children. Today's overweight child will become the obese young adult of tomorrow. And that obese young adult faces a lifetime of medical challenges, increasing medical care costs, decreased quality of life, and possibly a shortened lifespan. But remember, we're talking averages. This does not have to happen to you or your children or grandchildren. But preventing it means taking positive, proactive steps to avoid being the average. That's what this book is all about.

CALORIE RESTRICTION

Everyone knows that if you cut your calories you'll lose weight. But some research is now suggesting that if you continue on a lower-calorie, but healthy diet, you'll not only lose weight but you may gain a longer, healthier life as well. It's been known for years that if you restrict the calories in animals by 25-40 percent, but still feed them a nutritious diet, you can expand their lifespan significantly. They live 20-30 percent longer. And not only do they live longer, those extra years are healthy years as well. In fact, they are super-healthy years. Animals retain youthful coats and metabolisms, have better immune function, and are better able to fight off age-related problems like cancer and heart disease. This process called "calorie restriction," works throughout the animal kingdom, from the simplest organisms like yeast, to worms, fruit flies, and maybe even primates like monkeys.

Gerontologist Richard Weindruch of the University of Wisconsin at Madison studies calorie restriction in monkeys and has found that none of them develop diabetes over time compared to 50 percent of the monkeys fed a normal diet. The calorie restricted monkeys also have much lower body fat. Unfortunately they also have negative changes in bone density. Other labs have found decreases in libido, body temperature, and changes in menstrual cycles. What's more, a recent 25-year National Institutes of Health study published in *Nature* found no longevity benefit from calorie restriction. So, the jury's still out.

It turns out that through all these life forms we've mentioned, calorie restriction seems to stimulate a particular set of genes called NPT1 and SIR2. They're found in worms and they're found in humans. When these genes are stimulated they seem to help us live longer. Here is the supposed evolutionary logic: if food is scarce, then maybe the best thing is not to reproduce, but rather, work on surviving. As the body concentrates on survival during times of perceived stress and slows down it's normal aging process, it can, as a result, last longer so it can reproduce later when times are better.

THESE SO-CALLED LONGEVITY GENES NOT ONLY SLOW DOWN THE AGING PROCESS BUT THEY ALSO CHANGE THE METABOLIC RATE AND PROTECT THE CELLS FROM DAMAGE.

When these genes are activated, they stabilize chromosomes and DNA molecules, they promote DNA repair, and they regulate the genetic functions that control the activity of the cells of the body, all of which may help decrease cancer risk. They also switch on antioxidant and anti-inflammatory mechanisms in the cell and even cause some cancer cells to commit an organized suicide by a process called "apoptosis." In animal studies this has resulted in a reduction in risk factors for cardiac, diabetic, neurodegenerative diseases like

Alzheimer's and Parkinson's, and cancer.

Under normal conditions, these longevity genes are turned off. Some kind of environmental threat like extreme dieting or low calorie intake will activate them which may increase longevity.

Frankly, we don't know if calorie restriction works in humans. But whether you are a worm or a human, when you restrict calories your body perceives a threat. It thinks you're in the middle of a famine. It has the ability then to actually change the biochemistry of your body so that you slow down the "engine speed" of your metabolism. You also slow down the rate of aging in an effort to make it through what your body perceives as a dangerous time. Your body's trying to help you survive.

There's now a group of people in the United States that belong to something called "The Calorie Restriction Society." (www.crsociety.org) These are individuals that aren't waiting for the research on humans to come out. They eat good quality food but they limit their calorie intake to around 1400 calories a day. That's somewhere between a third and a half less than what the average American takes in.

Calorie restriction is usually a 30 percent reduction in calories that is slowly introduced over time. It results in decreased body fat which, in turn, results in a decrease of pro-inflammatory chemicals released from that body fat. Because members of the CRS understand nutrition and caloric density they still get to eat plenty of food but without a lot of calories. And the foods they eat are usually loaded with nutrition. Remember, if you know what you're doing, you can eat a lot of food without getting a lot of calories. An orange has a lot of nutrition but not many calories. A glass of orange juice has a lot of nutrition but a lot more calories. A potato has a lot of nutrition but not many calories. Potato chips have a lot more fat and calories even though it's the same food.

A GOOD GUIDELINE IS TO TRY TO EAT FOOD CLOSER TO THE WAY IT GROWS.

You're almost always going to get a better, more natural, less processed, lower calorie, more nutritious food that way. The point is you don't have to feel deprived on a reduced calorie diet if you get educated about nutrition. Nevertheless, it's going to be hard for the average person to cut their calories by 25-40 percent. What's more, following such a restricted diet seems to decrease your libido as well as your fertility. It may hurt your bone health as well.

Fortunately, a study recently published in the journal *Cell Metabolism* suggests that we might still be able to get the benefits of calorie restriction without having to completely dedicate ourselves to the effort. A pilot study using 19 human subjects found that three cycles of a five-day low calorie diet, given once per month, still resulted in a reduction of biomarkers for aging, cardiovascular disease, diabetes, and cancer.

> **SO, GOING ON A CALORIE-RESTRICTED REGIMEN NOW AND THEN, RATHER THAN FULL TIME, MAY STILL GIVE US BENEFITS.**

It would also be safer and a lot easier, too. Be watching for more developments in this area.

Just to clarify, calorie restriction doesn't simply mean eating less junk food or skipping dessert. It's reducing your calorie intake but still covering all your basic nutritional needs. In other words, you start eating good quality food, and only good quality food, but less than you normally would. By the way, it seems that it's the overall reduction in calories that works, not increasing or decreasing specific foods that contributes to longevity.

But we have a little problem here. A lot of people don't want to restrict their calories. Especially a lot of American people. Just look around. Americans are not known for calorie restriction. Wouldn't it be nice if we could come up with something that would stimulate these longevity genes without having to restrict our diets? Well it turns out there just might be something. It's something called "resveratol;" a natural substance you find in the skin of the red grape. Resveratrol targets the longevity genes and makes them more active, just like calorie restriction, without restricting calories! At least, that's the theory.

Researchers at Harvard Medical School added resveratrol to the feed of obese mice and found they became healthier and lived about 25 percent longer than similar mice that were not given the resveratrol. Unfortunately, normal weight mice that were given resveratrol did not live any longer. On the positive side though, the normal weight mice stayed much healthier as they got older; they had fewer cataracts, they were better coordinated, they had denser bones, and more flexible blood vessels. Resveratrol also seems to cause the SIRT1 gene to create new mitrochondria in the cell. This may account for the increased energy of older animals given resveratrol.

But, with humans, we have a challenge. You have to drink hundreds of bottles of red wine every day to get the equivalent of what was given to the mice. And we frankly don't know yet if the resveratrol supplements available at health food stores today actually have any biological effect. Maybe they do, maybe they don't. We also still don't know what an ideal dose would be.

Dr. David Sinclair of Harvard Medical School and other researchers have been working on developing a medication that would mimic the actions of resveratrol, without having to drink all that wine! To say the least, the research has had it's up's and down's. We still have a long way to go before we come up with a pill for humans.

So, in the meantime, do what you already know; continue to eat well and exercise and, if you smoke, stop. You don't want to die the day before the pill comes out.

5. START EATING MORE PLANT-BASED FOODS

We would do well today if we used terms like *vegan* and *vegetarian* less often. Not only do people have incorrect preconceived ideas of what those diets are like, but they also have political and social overtones as well. We'd be better off if we just focused on eating a more plant-based diet, period.

While people who eat that way have to be aware of their needs for vitamin B12, vitamin D, and protein, they stand to benefit greatly from eating differently than the average American.

People who eat more plant-based and less animal-based foods tend to weigh less and have less heart disease, diabetes, and cancer. They tend to live longer and healthier lives.

Here's some of the benefits of eating more fruits, vegetables, nuts, and whole grains:

WEIGHT CONTROL

Two out of three Americans are overweight. One child in three is overweight, as well. Research reported in *Nutrition Reviews* found that a vegetarian or vegan diet is very effective for weight loss.

One of the benefits of eating a more plant-based diet is that you tend to get more food but consume less calories. Since plant-based foods tend to have a lot more water and fiber content, they fill you up. That fiber helps keep your regular and can also lower blood cholesterol and blood sugar levels, too.

THOSE THAT EAT MORE PLANT-BASED FOODS SEEM TO HAVE AN EASIER TIME IN PREVENTING AGE-RELATED WEIGHT GAIN.

On the other hand, a study looking at data from the NHANES research found a positive association between meat consumption and obesity. In other words, the more meat consumed, the greater the likelihood of a problem with weight control.

PART 1: THE LONGEVITY RECIPE

New research also shows that a more plant-based diet seems to contribute to a healthier bacteria profile in your intestines. That, in turn, may help with weight control. Scientists recently reported in the *British Journal of Nutrition* that overweight women who took a probiotic supplement (of the bacteria *Lactobacillus rhamnosus*) lost twice as much weight and had an easier time of keeping it off compared to women taking a placebo.

A study done on twins found that those that were lean had a much greater diversity of gut bacteria than their overweight siblings. And recent research found that when bacteria from overweight humans was introduced into the intestines of normal weight mice, the mice became fat. When bacteria from lean humans was introduced into mice, the mice stayed lean. How do bacteria in your gut affect your waistline? Probably through a lot of mechanisms, but they seem to affect appetite, cravings, and how well your calories are absorbed and burned up. So what can you do? Foods that naturally contain bacteria, like yogurt, can help. Just make sure your brand says it contains "live active cultures," and that the sugar is low. Taking a probiotic supplement is also good; the kinds that require refrigeration are probably best. But what you normally eat every day can also greatly affect your gut bacteria profile. A more plant-based, less processed food diet tends to give you a healthier bacteria population that will probably contribute to easier weight control. Stay tuned, we still have a lot to learn.

HEART DISEASE PREVENTION

In a study at Harvard that followed 110,000 people for 14 years, it was observed that, compared to those who only ate one and a half servings per day, those who consumed an average of eight servings of fruits and vegetables a day were 30 percent less likely to have a heart attack or stroke. And remember, a serving is often just a half a cup.

In his Lifestyle Heart Trial, Dr. Dean Ornish found that heart patients that followed his plant-based diet actually experienced a degree of reversal of their atherosclerosis after one year. That's amazing! We never knew until recently that you could actually reverse the disease known as "hardening of the arteries." We thought the best you could do was to keep the disease from getting worse.

His diet included about 10 percent of the calories from fat, about 20 percent from protein, and about 70 percent from complex whole-grain carbohydrates. And while that is a very low-fat diet, the Lyon Diet Heart Study also found protection from heart attacks and premature death in those that ate a more liberal Mediterranean style type diet that included a higher fat intake and fish.

One in three Americans currently suffers from high blood pressure which can increase their risk for heart disease and stroke. A great deal of research indicates that a diet that includes lots of fruits and vegetables can help lower that blood pressure.

DECREASED DIABETES

About 95 percent of diabetics today are type-2 diabetics; the kind that is entirely lifestyle related. Since obesity is the primary contributing factor to the development of type-2 diabetes, and since it's much easier to maintain a healthy weight on a more plant-based diet, it just makes sense that eating more fruits, vegetables, and whole grain breads and cereals can dramatically decrease your risk of ever developing diabetes in the first place. Researchers have found that vegetarians have only about half the risk of developing diabetes compared to non-vegetarians.

A plant-based diet also seems to be beneficial by improving insulin sensitivity and decreasing insulin resistance. A diet based on fruits, vegetables, and whole grains cannot only help prevent diabetes, but it may help those with the disease to more successfully manage it, too.

CANCER REDUCTION

A plant-based diet may prevent or slow the growth of certain cancers including those of the breast, prostate, colon, and cervix. It may also help with preventing or slowing BPH, benign prostatic hypertrophy. Since plant foods contain hundreds of natural anti-aging phytochemicals, they can help the body improve its own natural cancer defenses.

According to the American Cancer Society, the average consumption of meat in the Western diet, specifically red meat like beef, pork, and processed meat like bacon, seems to increase the risk of cancer. In addition to it's saturated fat content, meat contains a certain kind of unique iron called "heme iron;" a combination of iron and a protein called "heme." It's this heme iron that contributes to the formation of nitrosamines in the large intestine which, in turn, seems to increase cancer risk.

Many of the long-lived healthy people around the world never had much access to meat; primarily because it's usually so expensive. While meat is a good source of protein, protein has been oversold in the United States. If you're over 19 years of age you can get by quite nicely with somewhere between 50-80 g of protein per day. That's very easy to get. And you don't have to eat meat to get your protein. In addition to chicken and fish, non-animal sources of protein include beans, whole grains, peanut butter, soy foods, and nuts.

We know that those who have a more plant-based diet have much better health outcomes than the average meat-eating American. We also now know that you can get a lot of the same benefits from eating what's called the Mediterranean diet. The details of that are coming up later.

A BETTER ENVIRONMENT

McDonalds sells 75 hamburgers every second of every hour, every single day. We Americans eat 50 billion burgers a year. Our meat-based food system requires more energy, land, and water resources than we can sustain over the long-term. The US population of 320 million is expected to double in the next eighty years. Our children and grandchildren may be forced to eat a healthier, more plant-based diet, simply because of a lack of resources. It takes about 2500 gallons of water to produce one pound of beef. One pound of wheat only requires 25 gallons. The US Geological Survey says that 40 percent of freshwater used in the US goes to irrigate feed crops for livestock. Only about 13 percent is used for such human activities as flushing toilets, washing cars, watering lawns, and taking showers. We could feed a lot more humans if some of the water used for livestock crops went for human crops. With water becoming harder to come by, especially in certain regions, a more plant-based diet could help protect this valuable resource.

According to the Nature Conservancy, one football field of rainforest is destroyed every second of every day! Much of that is used to raise livestock. With that rainforest goes hundreds of plant and animal species, never to be replaced again. What's more, the rainforests play a vital role in the world's oxygen supply.

The meat industry is the number one producer of methane gas on the planet. That methane gas traps heat in the atmosphere and can contribute to a rise in the earth's temperature. Yes, I know there's a lot of controversy out there about global warming, the rainforest, and related topics. But methane produced from cattle is much more powerful of a greenhouse gas than carbon dioxide. We could drive more cars if we would eat less cows.

6. EAT MORE NUTS!

For years nuts have been on the list of foods that dieters had to avoid. In just one cup of cashews you get 56 grams of fat and almost 700 calories. One cup of peanuts will cost you 72 grams of fat and over 800 calories! I don't about you, but I personally can go thru a cup of cashews without much effort. While it's true that they're high in calories and fat, it's that fat that's now making researchers take a second look. It turns out that nuts are not only loaded with vitamins, minerals, fiber, and other healthy substances, but the fat they contain is generally pretty good for you, too. Researchers have discovered that a lot of healthy people eat nuts as part of their regular diet. Since they seem to be so important for a healthy, long life, let's spend some time on the details you need to know.

NUTS FOR YOUR HEART

Nuts seem to be especially good for your heart. Remember, you only get cholesterol from animal foods and since nuts are plants they are naturally cholesterol free. Recently, Harvard researchers looked at more than 86,000 nurses over 14 years and found that those that ate more than about a half-cup of nuts per week were about a third less likely to develop heart disease or have a heart attack than women who didn't. Another group at Harvard found the same results in a group of 22,000 male physicians that they followed for 12 years.

> **THE IOWA WOMEN'S HEALTH STUDY FOUND THAT THOSE WOMEN WHO ATE NUTS OR SEEDS FOUR OR MORE TIMES A WEEK WERE 40 PERCENT LESS LIKELY TO DIE FROM HEART DISEASE THAN THOSE WOMEN WHO ATE NONE.**

And in a review of 16 studies, researchers at Penn State University said that eating an ounce of nuts more than five times a week could reduce heart disease risk by 25-39 percent. The great news is that nuts seem to have this beneficial effect on everyone; young and old, male and female.

Some studies have shown that nuts can also increase your good HDL cholesterol. A recent study in South Africa has also shown specifically how much the various types of nuts can lower your bad LDL cholesterol. For example, if you eat about an ounce and a half each day for four weeks you can expect a reduction of about 6½ percent from peanuts, 7½ percent from walnuts, about 8 percent from almonds, and about 13½ percent from pecans. Please note, that's pecans, not pecan pie.

Do you like walnuts? Humans have been eating them since about 7000 B.C.. That's a lot of walnuts! Because they kind of look like the brain, they were used during the Renaissance to treat head aliments. Today, about 99 percent of them come from California which also supplies about 2/3 of what the world consumes.

Most nuts are good sources of the healthy monounsaturated fats. However, walnuts are unique in that they contain high amounts of polyunsaturated fat. A recent study showed that walnuts, which help lower cholesterol like other nuts, may particularly be good for your arteries. Researchers found that walnuts even improved an already healthy Mediterranean type diet. When they replaced some of the healthy monounsaturated fats like that found in olive oil with an equal number of calories from walnuts, the elasticity of the subjects arteries improved. This allows for an easier flow of blood through those arteries. That's especially important in possibly decreasing high blood pressure risk. Walnuts have an especially high level of something called alpha-linolenic acid and a form of vitamin E, both of which can be good for your heart. The Food and Drug Administration has said that, in addition to eating a diet low in saturated fat, eating just 1½ ounces of walnuts a day may help decrease your risk of heart disease. By the way, that's about 15, half-walnuts.

Want some more good news? Walnuts are also a rich source of natural substances called "phytosterols" which block some of the cholesterol you eat from being absorbed in your intestine. Walnuts may look like your brain, but they're good for your heart!

BRAZIL NUTS, ALMONDS, AND CASHEWS, OH MY!

Brazil nuts are an incredibly rich source of the mineral selenium. Just one Brazil nut gives you all you need of this hard to get important trace mineral for the entire day. If a man eats two or three of them a day he takes in the amount of selenium that's been shown in some studies to lower the risk of prostate cancer.

Almonds are a nutritional superstar. They have

more fiber, calcium, vitamin E, and the B vitamin riboflavin than any other nut. Just one serving gives you half of the recommended vitamin E you need for the entire day. They've got magnesium, potassium, phosphorous, iron, and the good monounsaturated fats, too. And people like them! Did you know that instead of rice, Italians shower newlyweds with almonds? In India, pregnant women are told to eat almonds everyday. And at the end of a Greek wedding reception, guests are given a small bundle of candy-coated almonds.

Researchers at the University of Illinois at Chicago found that almonds given to mice with an Alzheimer's-like disease for four months did better on a memory test. What's more, the diet also reduced the number of Alzheimer deposits found in their brains. And it didn't take much to see these results; just the human equivalent of about a handful a day. Of course, this doesn't prove that almonds will help humans prevent Alzheimer's, but it's certainly suggestive knowing what we do know about the other good benefits that come from almonds.

You could start eating a handful of almonds everyday, couldn't you? And remember a serving of almonds is just that, a handful. That comes to an ounce or about 23 almonds. It's also a ¼ cup, an empty tin of Altoids mints, or two wells of an ice-cube tray. You get the idea.

At Christmas time you might sing about chestnuts roasting on an open fire. But that may be about all you know about them. Chestnuts are produced once a year, in the fall. We used to grow a lot of them here in the US until about a hundred years ago when a fungus wiped out most of our industry. Today they come from Europe and Asia for the most part. Now if you have to watch your fat, chestnuts are for you! They're the lowest of all the nuts when it comes to fat and calories. Once again, remember that the fat from nuts is not bad for you, but it's sure easy to take in a lot of calories from nuts if you're not careful.

Fortunately, you really don't have to be careful when it comes to chestnuts. They only get about 1 percent of their calories from fat whereas many others in the nut family come in at 70 percent or more. Unfortunately, they also don't have the fiber or protein you find in most other nuts either. Surprisingly, chestnuts are the only nuts to have vitamin C. While you can eat them raw, they're usually baked, roasted, or boiled to bring out their natural sweetness. Look for those that feel heavy and hard and are a shiny brown in color. If you want to try your hand at the old tradition of roasting chestnuts, cut an "x" into the flat side of the shells with a sharp knife. Just cut through the very thin shell, but not into the nut itself. Bake those for about 15 minutes in a 400 degree oven until they've browned. To make it easy on yourself you can buy them already peeled in cans or peeled and roasted in jars.

Of course, the best tasting nut of all is the cashew. I don't care what you say; I don't care what anyone says. It just is. Cashews are the best! I like peanut butter, but I really LOVE cashews. The flavor, the aroma, the slightly sweet taste. Yum!

CASHEWS ARE ALSO THE BEST OF THE NUTS WHEN IT COMES TO THEIR COPPER AND ZINC CONTENT.

I'm no longer low in copper or zinc. I suggest you try adding some cashews to your peanut butter. Mmmmm!

Nuts are rich in magnesium and fiber which can help control insulin and blood sugar levels. It's not surprising, therefore, that some research has suggested that nuts or peanut butter consumed as part of your diet may help reduce your risk of type-2 diabetes. Magnesium is also involved in the functioning of your heart, muscles, nerves, bones, energy production, and blood clotting. Many Americans, especially the elderly, don't get enough magnesium since they generally consume less of it and their body doesn't absorb it as well as when they were younger.

NUTS MAY ALSO HELP DECREASE YOUR RISK OF DEVELOPING GALLSTONES, TOO.

In the Nurses Health study, researchers followed some 80,000 women for 20 years and found that those who ate five or more ounces of nuts or nut butters per week were 23 percent less likely to need surgery for gallstones. The guess is that nuts may decrease bile secretion and cholesterol production and thereby reduce the risk of stone formation.

Of the nuts, almonds, hazelnuts, macadamias, pecans, and pistachios contain the greatest amounts of the good monounsaturated fats. Peanuts are also a good source and additionally contain our old friend "resveratrol," the substance also found in grapes and red wine that seems to be good for heart health. What's more, peanuts have the most protein of the nuts. If you're trying to cut down on animal fats like meats and cheese, nuts offer you a great, healthy alternative without

PART 1: THE LONGEVITY RECIPE 61

compromising on nutrition.

By the way, peanuts are not actually nuts. They're legumes, like dried beans. They grow underground in pods as opposed to other nuts like almonds and pecans which grow on trees. Nevertheless, they have a similar healthy nutritional profile as the rest of the nuts and they're often used in similar ways in recipes. And soy nuts are also not actually nuts, either; they're roasted soybeans. You can get them either dry-roasted or fried. Get the dry-roasted, they make a good snack and they have lots of soy protein and those good-for-you plant compounds called "isoflavones." Watch for the added salt, though. If you can get them without, that's better.

So remember, peanuts are not actually nuts. Soy nuts are not actually nuts. Technically, Brazil nuts and cashews are also not nuts, they're seeds. And donuts are not actually nuts, either. Although you can get donuts with nuts.

PEANUT BUTTER

After I tell people about the high fat content of nuts and peanuts, one of the next questions they often ask is "well, what about peanut butter?" So, where does peanut butter come from? ....Peanuts. So, yes peanuts are high in fat; peanut butter is high in fat. That's no problem if you eat a tablespoon or so. But a lot of people just sit there with a spoon and eat it out of the jar. Peanut butter is a good thing, but it's real easy to get too much of a good thing.

Now if you like your peanut butter real smooth and creamy like I do, you've often had to consume those nasty partially hydrogenated oils along with it. Not only do they make it easier to spread, but the peanut butter also lasts a lot longer without going bad. Did you ever notice that you don't usually have to refrigerate most peanut butters? It's those partially hydrogenated oils that do the trick. But remember, those partially hydrogenated oils is where we get trans fats from. And they're bad news. But the good news is that the government has recently mandated that manufacturers now remove trans fats from all their products. They're replacing them with palm and palm kernel oil. And while they add some saturated fat, that's not as bad as the trans fats they replaced. Plus, you'll still get a nice smooth peanut butter that won't separate. But, once again, remember that the suggested serving size for peanut butter is two tablespoons. And that's two level tablespoons; not how much you can balance on two tablespoons.

Now if you're a purist, and want to avoid palm

and palm kernel oil too, just buy plain natural peanut butter. The ingredient listing is usually pretty short. Peanuts. No salt, no sugar, no hydrogenated fat, no palm or palm kernel oil, nothing added or taken away. These jars are usually the ones with the oil floating on top. Peanuts and peanut butter naturally have about two to three grams of saturated fat per serving. But that's in there naturally. Don't worry about that.

> **YES, SOME BRANDS OF NATURAL PEANUT BUTTER WILL HAVE SOME SALT OR SUGAR ADDED BUT IT'S USUALLY NOT MUCH AND IT DOES MAKE FOR A BETTER TASTING PRODUCT.**

Have you noticed these low-fat peanut butters in the grocery store? They really don't help you much since the calories they saved by reducing the fat are usually added back in with the sugar they add to improve the flavor. For example, reduced-fat peanut butter only has 12 grams of fat per serving compared to regular peanut butter's 17 grams. I like that. But the calories are still the same. I'm not that impressed.

Something that does impress me, however, are these "whipped peanut butters." By whipping air into peanut butter you can make it a lot easier to spread. That's nice and it also means you're getting less fat per serving since you're getting more air. It's the same way they decrease fat and calories in some margarines; they simply whip air into them. And unlike those reduced fat peanut butters, this really makes a difference. As we said, regular peanut butter has about 17 grams of fat per serving and 190 calories. But whipped just has 12 grams of fat and 140 calories. Now it's true, they're charging you about the same amount and you're technically getting less food because of the whipped-in air, but this is still a legitimate way for you to eat your peanut butter and cut down on both fat and calories. The bottom line, don't bother with those reduced fat peanut butters, but the whipped peanut butters are worth a try.

It's estimated that about one out of every one hundred Americans is allergic to nuts. The most common sensitivities are to peanuts and walnuts. Symptoms can include hives, itchy mouth, wheezing, difficulty breathing, diarrhea and vomiting and, in severe cases, even anaphylactic shock. Of course, if that's you, all this good news about the health benefits of nuts doesn't get you very excited. You've also had to become a very good label reader. Products in the supermarket, of course, list their ingredients but now also will tell you even if they've been produced in a plant that also processes nuts. If you can't do peanut butter, don't forget you have lots of other nut butter options available. If you can handle them, everything from almond, hazelnut, cashew, soy, macadamia, and sesame seed butter can be good choices and give you some variety, too. The same rules about moderation with peanut butter apply to these other nut butters as well.

NUTS AND YOUR WAISTLINE

If you're watching you calories, remember that macadamia nuts contain the most calories and fat per serving. They come in at 205 calories and 21 grams of fat per ounce. On the other hand, an ounce of chestnuts contain the least with just 70 calories and less than one gram of fat.

Just how many nuts do you get in an ounce? Here's the numbers: 6-8 Brazil nuts, 16-18 cashews, 18-20 pecan halves, 10-12 macadamias, 45-47 pistachios, 18-20 hazelnuts, 150-157 pine nuts, 8-11 walnut halves, and 20-24 almonds.

Have you ever seen the term "dry roasted" used on a jar of nuts? What does that mean? Basically just that they weren't "oil roasted," which is the other option. In other words, fried. The manufacturers simply roast them in a little peanut oil instead of roasting them plain. If it doesn't say "dry roasted," you can assume they were fried. Cocktail peanuts are usually fried. The important thing to remember, however, is that since nuts are naturally so high in fat to begin with, their preparation method doesn't really affect the fat content or calories that much. Yes, dry roasted is better, but not by much.

STUDIES HAVE SHOWN THAT WHEN PEOPLE ADD NUTS TO THEIR DIET, THEY USUALLY DON'T GAIN WEIGHT.

True, nuts have lots of calories. But apparently when people add moderate amounts of nuts to their regular intake, they seem to handle it without weight gain. Don't miss that, when people add *moderate* amounts they don't gain weight. A study at Purdue University looked at women who added 344 calories worth of almonds to their intake everyday. They did not purposely cut back on their intake of other foods and yet at the end of ten weeks they didn't gain any weight. Other studies have found the same thing with peanuts and almonds. It may be that people unconsciously decrease their calories from other foods to make up the difference. Some research has shown that not all the fat in whole nuts is absorbed by the body. It's estimated that somewhere between 4-17 percent goes through the body undigested. Whatever the reason, the good news is that the research shows you can add a handful of nuts to your regular diet and not pay the price! Again, that's a handful, not a jar full!

But you can have too much of a good thing. A study done at Loma Linda University gave eighty-one middle-aged men and women about 2½ ounces of almonds a day for six months. They did not give them any advice on eating less or more of any other foods. At the end of six months, the women only gained one-fifth of a pound, but the men gained an average of a pound and a half. Obviously, if that continued, that could be a problem. But to be fair, they were eating 2½ ounces. That's about twice of what we're recommending. There may be a limit to how many nuts you can eat, before the calories do start to kick in.

NUTS TO YOU!

Don't think of nuts as you would other snacks. We're learning more and more about how good they really are for you. So eat more nuts as you decrease snacks like cookies, crackers, and chips.

You'll be improving the quality of you daily nutrition without adding extra calories. And because nuts are high in fiber and healthy fat, they tend to satisfy and fill you up; a light snack of some nuts before a meal can actually help you eat less. So just be aware of the amounts you're eating. It doesn't take many nuts to give you some real health benefits. And instead of just sitting down with a bowlful, use them as part of a meal. You can chop them up and add them to fruit and regular salads, oatmeal, pancakes, and yogurt.

Regardless of what kind of nuts you're eating, it's always better to eat the unsalted kind if you need to control your sodium intake. There are plenty of those available now. And if you don't like the salt-free varieties, you can also get the "lightly salted" ones that only have about half as much sodium as the regular kind. And as we said, most nuts are also high in fiber, magnesium, and potassium which all may help to additionally lower blood pressure.

So, surprise, nuts are good for you! Yes, it's still true that Americans are eating a lot of fat; and a lot of the wrong kind. But we now know it's not only how much fat you eat, but what kind of fat you eat that matters. By eating less saturated animal fats like those found in meats, cheese, and whole dairy products, and replacing that fat with the kind found in nuts, you can still eat foods that will taste good, be satisfying, and be good for you, too. So…nuts to you!

7. LEARN TO HANDLE STRESS

Stress is a killer. Scientists have recently learned that stress seems to be related to dangerous inflammation that's often found throughout the body. That inflammation can, in turn, be related to the development of many long-term diseases like atherosclerosis, Alzheimer's, and diabetes. It may be that handling stress can help keep this inflammation under long-term control and minimize those diseases.

Part of handling that stress is the ability to know what's really important in life. That viewpoint helps us deal with the daily aggravations and keep things in perspective.

A lot of stress is self-inflicted. Have you noticed, some people are their own worst enemy? There's an old joke about a clean desk being a sign of a sick mind. The reality, however, is than disorganization is a major source of stress. This may come as no surprise, but it seems that conscientious people tend to live longer. A researcher at the University of California at Riverside found that children who were conscientious young in life had the greatest life expectancy. They were the ones that could be depended upon to do their homework and put their bicycles away without being reminded.

As you might guess, conscientious people think things through before doing them. They often have more order in their life and have ambitious long-term goals. People that are not conscientious tend to jump in with both feet and worry about the consequences later; they're more impulsive and less organized. They drive motorcycles without helmets and they don't remember to take their vitamins. The conscientious may not seem to be as much "fun" as their more risk-taking peers, but they tend to outlive them.

By the way, researchers at the State University of New York at Buffalo found that everything else being equal, people with a pet have lower stress levels than those who don't. People who exercise also have lower stress hormones. So go take your dog for a walk.

Remember that part of stress is perception. What's stressful to one person may be a common everyday routine for another person. Most people would agree, it's not what happens to you, it's how you react to what happens to you.

> **DR. LEONARD POON, THE DIRECTOR OF THE UNIVERSITY OF GEORGIA GERONTOLOGY CENTER FOUND THAT 100-YEAR-OLDS EXHIBIT FOUR STRESS COPING MECHANISMS.**

First, they tend to be more dominant. They want to have things their way and they don't like being pushed around. Number two, many tend to be somewhat suspicious; they don't necessarily take things at face value. They tend to question an issue and think it through. Thirdly, they tend to be practical, not idealistic. And finally, they tend to be more relaxed. They're strong characters but they're also flexible.

Those people that live a long healthy life demonstrate the ability to "roll with the punches." It's not that they avoid the stresses of life but that they have the ability to respond to them deliberatively and efficiently. They also have the ability to snap back from losses, even the deaths of family and friends. They mourn appropriately, but then they get on with life. That has to do, in part, with their ability to develop and maintain relationships, which, as we said earlier, seems to be vitally important to health. They remain flexible in their dealings with other people and society and they can integrate new things and ideas into their life. They can handle everyday problem solving and they also stay in touch with the outside world, usually with people younger than them by a generation or more. A good sense of humor seems to be common in healthy older people as well.

A lot of people deal with stress by using tobacco. Unfortunately, the short-term stress relief they get just brings on more stress from related health problems in the long run. Tobacco increases your risk of heart attack and atherosclerosis, chronic bronchitis, emphysema, and cancer. But, of course, you already knew that. Fortunately, most Americans don't smoke anymore. But about 20 percent of adults in this country still do. Let's face it, if you've been smoking for years you may actually like smoking. But about a half a million people die from smoking related causes every year just in the US. Every year. 500,000 people. There's nothing to like about that. We have medicines now that can take away your addiction to cigarettes. They're not nicotine replacements, and they're not perfect, but they get to the cause of why you can't stop. Ask your doctor about them. Above everything else, tobacco will keep you from having a healthy, long life.

A POSITIVE ATTITUDE

Related to your ability to handle stress is your attitude. Is your glass always half empty or half full? We see a good sense of optimism in most people who live long healthy lives. Surprisingly, research indicates that you seem to get a better increase in longevity from an optimistic viewpoint than you do even from lowering blood cholesterol levels.

Baseball great Satchel Paige is quoted as saying "How old would you be if you didn't know how old you are?" Your attitude about growing older may, in fact, affect how you do grow older. A study done at the National Institute on Aging found that 40 and 50-year-old people who have a negative attitude toward aging tend to age worse than those who have a positive view about it. It appears that those who fight the aging process seem to do better than those who just passively accept it.

But as we said earlier, the reality about old age

is that the news is good. Only one out of every four individuals 85 years of age and over currently suffers from a severe impairment. Having the right attitude about aging is mostly up to you. Some things that help include exercising, getting a hobby, remaining socially active in something that gets you out of the house, and proactively working on a positive attitude.

Consider this. While the risk of Alzheimer's does goes up as we age, dementia is not inevitable. You also don't have to end up in a nursing home. Only about 30 percent of people who are aged 100 are both mentally and physically impaired. Another 40 percent have some limitations in vision, mental function or mobility but they still do well. And the final third really don't have any restrictions to speak of at all.

Keep in mind that today there are about 80,000 hundred-year-olds just in the United States. 80,000! A third of them with no impairments is a lot of well functioning centenarians walking around right now.

Optimists tend to expect positive outcomes in their life and they believe that they have the ability to accomplish what they set out to do. A big part of that optimism is having a sense of gratitude and letting go of grievances. Mayo Clinic found that those scoring the highest on a pessimism scale were 20 percent more likely to die prematurely than the optimistic. Pessimists tend to develop "can't win" attitudes and are less likely to take positive care of themselves, get medical help, eat well, and avoid cigarettes. Pessimism may actually harm your immune system as well. Pessimists are more likely to develop colds. In cancer patients, optimists tend to have better long-term results.

THE HUGE GOVERNMENT STUDY CALLED "THE WOMEN'S HEALTH INITIATIVE" FOUND A RELATIONSHIP BETWEEN CYNICISM AND HOSTILITY AND A HIGHER RISK OF CANCER AND HEART DISEASE.

Anger and hostility don't do your body any good; especially the face-reddening, furniture-pounding kind. It can cause cortisol, adrenaline, and other body chemicals to thicken your blood and make it more likely to clot. Your risk of having a heart attack can double following one of these fits of anger.

If you're consistently pessimistic it may be that you're that way for a reason. It could be that you got the short end of the stick too many times in life. Bad things do, indeed, happen to good people. Life, as you probably know, is not fair. But again, it's not just what happens to you, but how you think about it!

YOUR LIFE OUTLOOK STYLE, POSITIVE OR NEGATIVE, SEEMS TO STAY THE SAME THROUGHOUT LIFE, UNLESS YOU WORK TO CHANGE IT.

But, if you decide to, you'll probably need assistance to change your way of thinking, especially the older you get. Learning the skills to make the best out of both negative and positive events in life takes effort. Some counselors believe something called "cognitive therapy" can do the trick. You can visit www.academyofct.org or www.abct.org for a nationwide referral service. With "positive psychology" people can learn to be optimistic and more happy at any age. A support group, medication for depression, or finding a pain clinic may help you get started in the right direction.

How do you become optimistic? Some people are just naturally born that way. But it's not easy for a lot of us, especially if we're regularly bombarded with the daily stressors of modern-day life. Things don't always turn out right. Nevertheless, count

PART 1: THE LONGEVITY RECIPE

your blessings. Look at what you really do have. Yes there are some people out there that have it better than you. But, regardless of where you are in American society, if you compare yourself to the average human you are far, far better off than most people who have ever lived on this planet. That's a fact.

By the way, research continues to show that money does not make you optimistic or buy happiness. As long as the basic financial needs of life are covered, money does little to affect how happy you are. On the other hand, a conscious effort to dwell on the good things of life and positive long-term memories can affect your daily mood. Work on consciously becoming more aware of all the blessings in your life.

But don't get too optimistic. You may start to think that you're immune to any problems. Optimism that gets out of hand can deceive you into thinking that you can break all the rules of health and still come out smelling like a rose. A healthy dose of optimism balanced with a realistic view of life is the best approach.

8. REALIZE THAT THERE IS A SPIRITUAL DIMENSION TO LIFE

Many people around the world today still believe that there's more to life than just the physical dimension of the five senses. Spirituality can take many forms and doesn't necessarily have to mean organized religion. In general, it usually reflects having a sense of something greater than oneself and a realization of the meaning of one's existence.

While not all research shows a protective effect from regular church attendance, the vast majority does. A study published in the journal *Demography* looked at 20,000 Americans and found that whites who attended church lived about seven years longer than their non-churchgoing counterparts. African-Americans lived 14 years longer than those who did not attend church. Another study that looked at over 3600 people found that those who attended a religious service at least once a month decreased their death rate by about one third from those who did not attend as often. A study funded by the National Institutes of Health that looked at 34,000 people over a period of 12 years found that those who went to church frequently decreased their death rate by about 20 percent.

Being part of a religious network, of course, is also a way to stay socially connected. For many people, it's their most important social support group. That social support may encourage them to practice prevention and get earlier treatment for health problems. People who go to church on a regular basis tend to follow healthier behaviors as well. They're less likely to smoke, abuse drugs or alcohol, and are more physically active. Those that acknowledge a spiritual side of life have lower risks of depression, suicide, high blood pressure, cardiovascular disease, and cancer. Their immune system seems to function better as well.

Coming to the realization that the world does not revolve around you after all, and realizing that you're part of something bigger, seems to significantly help with stress reduction, self-reflection, and overall better physical health. Believing that God is ultimately in control takes away a lot of stress and anxiety that people might otherwise put on themselves. It gives hope for the future and a purpose to life.

Regardless if it's eventually determined that religious or spiritual faith is an actual cause of better health, or simply results in better health, the benefits remain the same. People who have a spiritual/religious dimension to their lives seem to be healthier.

9. STOP BLAMING YOUR PARENTS

Obviously, genetics plays some role in how long you live. For example, brothers of centenarians are seventeen times as likely to live to 100 as are people without centenarians in the family. Sisters of centenarians are 8.5 times as likely to live to 100. Children of centenarians in their 70's and 80's have a 60 percent reduced risk of heart disease, stroke and diabetes.

Experts say that the average person is born with strong enough longevity genes to live to about 85. People who take appropriate preventive steps may add 10 years to that. That, of course, is the point of this book. Those that make it to 100 and over can usually thank their family for some good genes.

A study done in Sweden of identical twins showed that about 30 percent of longevity is genetically determined. However, their ultimate lifespan, like everyone else's, really was determined by their lifestyle habits. If it was all genetics, identical twins should live about the same length of life, but they don't. They often have different health and sickness experiences and ultimately die at different ages.

A healthy lifestyle will maximize your genetic potential. That's good news. You can't do much about your genetics, yet, but you can improve your lifestyle. Your genetics do seem to be more important to your longevity, however, if your parents lived past age 90 or if they died prematurely from disease. Genetics probably influences an individual's ability to overcome a disease or injury and also effects how much of an organ is necessary for its continued performance. For example, an autopsy on a 103-year-old man who had no signs of Alzheimer's still showed the physical evidence of it in his brain. Because of his good genetics, he had enough excess reserve of his brain function that he could still think properly even though the disease was present.

A major discovery in the early 1990's was that there are just several single genes that control the aging process. We never knew till then that aging was so closely regulated. If we can learn how to control those aging genes, we should be able to have a dramatic effect on both the quality and quantity of human life.

These longevity genes are collectively referred to as "sirtuins." It turns out that all organisms from the lowest simple yeast up to us complicated humans have them. People that live very long lives and in relatively good health may simply have sirtuin genes that are much more effective and efficient than the average person's. Probably by a number of different mechanisms, their genes are much better at fighting off disease and maintaining health. We may not understand all the ways that the sirtuin genes affect human longevity for many years yet, but their mechanism is not near as important as the fact that we've identified the genes themselves and that they do affect our longevity. That's been a major discovery.

Here's just a quick anatomy lesson for you. A chromosome is an organized structure of DNA and protein that is found in the nucleus of every one of our cells. The chromosome contains many genes, regulatory elements and other nucleotide sequences. The chromosomes form an X or Y configuration. At the very end of each one of the legs of the chromosome are something called "telomeres." They act to keep the chromosomes from unraveling or degrading. Telomeres on our chromosomes would be similar to the plastic tip on the end of a shoelace. Every time a cell divides the telomeres of its daughter cells become shorter and shorter. That shortening, by the way, can also come from stress and other negative lifestyle influences.

MOST CELLS HAVE A SORT OF BUILT-IN COUNTER THAT LIMITS THE NUMBER OF TIMES THEY CAN DIVIDE.

After about 100 replications the telomeres become so short that the cell can no longer reproduce. So the shorter the telomeres, the older the cell.

Recently, researchers measured the length of telomeres in the white blood cells of 2400 twins and found that the most physically active twins had significantly longer telomeres than the twins that were least active. The most active twins averaged about 30 minutes of activity a day. One guess is that activity helps decrease body inflammation and oxidative stress. Both of those are known to shorten telomere length. This may be one way that exercise helps you live longer and healthier.

> **WE HAVE ALSO RECENTLY DISCOVERED A TELOMERE-PRESERVING ENZYME CALLED "TELOMERASE" THAT ALLOWS THE CELL TO KEEP ON LIVING AND REPRODUCING.**

It's possible that telomerase is one more of the mechanisms by which the sirtuin genes have their effect on longevity. A study done in men by Dr. Dean Ornish showed that a healthy lifestyle increases this telomerase. The men in the study improved their diet, reduced stress, and exercised moderately. And their telomerase went up. The activity of disease-preventing genes also increased and some disease-promoting genes actually shut down. The ones that shut down were those specifically involved in promoting prostate and breast cancer.

We used to think that human aging was pre-programmed into each one of us. We thought it was just a normal part of the ongoing development of the human body. We now know that's not true.

For the most part, it appears that human aging results when the body's normal repair and maintenance mechanisms, controlled by our genes, simply don't work as well as they did when we were younger. We're not really programmed to get old, we get old because we lose the ability to repair the day-to-day damage that happens from life.

Currently almost all medical effort goes into treating diseases. But the research that discovered the sirtuins, the longevity genes, is now suggesting that we may actually be able to address the aging process itself that contributes to these diseases. There may be many processes that cause aging but the sirtuins is where we should still intervene. We now understand that there is a single intervention that addresses the fundamental issue of aging itself. We now understand that aging is much more subject to modification than was ever thought in the past.

We aren't necessarily talking about making old people live longer but, rather, about helping people stay younger as they get older. That's an important difference. We may, indeed, be able to help people live longer lives but, more importantly, it now seems that we may also be able to improve the quality of those years as well. Remember, the best thing in life is to die young, as late as you possibly can.

Don't count on any miraculous scientific discovery to soon defeat America's big killers. Not only is that a huge undertaking that's been going on for decades, a study published by top scientists recently in *Health Affairs* reveals that the best return on time and dollar investment is, once again, in addressing the aging process itself. Since it is the aging process that is the underlying cause of most major diseases, we will receive far greater benefit from addressing that issue rather than continuing to attack individual health problems like heart disease and cancer. For example, the study showed that even modestly slowing the aging process would result in a five percent increase in healthy, non-disabled adults 65 and over every year from the years 2030 to 2060. While it may not sound like much, just five percent is still a lot of otherwise sick people who now stay healthy and in need of a lot less medical care.

The study also revealed that the current model of trying to conquer individual diseases would result in almost no improvement in quality of life. An older population that stays healthier longer is not only a gold-mine of medical care savings, but the goal of most all of us; a long life with quality of life.

PART 1: THE LONGEVITY RECIPE

The very smart people at Google—yes, that Google—have recently created a new biotech company called Calico to research some of these very fundamental aging issues. What they ultimately discover may make even the success of their search engine pale by comparison.

So, if you're able, hang on for about twenty or so more years, until gene therapy becomes practical. Then you'll be able to take advantage of real longevity improvements. This finally could change the basic medical model from treatment to prevention. In the meantime, what you learn here will help you have a better quality of life until that day comes.

Here's the bottom line on genetics as of now.

MOST OF US HAVE THE GENETIC POTENTIAL TO LIVE INTO OUR LATE 80S OR EARLY 90S.

On our own, and until genetic therapy becomes practical, we can't do anything to lengthen that genetic potential. But the wrong lifestyle decisions can definitely cut it short. That's what most people do. But remember, to reach your maximum lifespan potential it's 70 percent lifestyle and only 30 percent genetics. Those people that make it to 100 and over have inherited better genes and have lived a healthy lifestyle. But a poor lifestyle can keep them from reaching their genetic potential, too. Your personal health decisions are VERY important.

10. BEAT THE TWO BIG KILLERS

Life expectancy has only increased significantly in the last two hundred years or so. But it's not that people are living that much longer, contrary to what many people think. George Washington and our other founding fathers lived well into their 70's and 80's. The difference is that scientific and medical advances have dramatically cut the deaths of babies and young children. So when you average the death of an 80-year-old with a baby who died at birth, the life expectancy averages out to only 40. But if you can keep those babies and children alive because of better hygiene, better sanitation, and antibiotics, then the average lifespan goes up.

Two thousand years ago the average lifespan was

PART 1: THE LONGEVITY RECIPE 89

22. During the 17th century it was 35. By the year 1908 it was 49. Today the average lifespan for a woman is 81 and the average for a man, about 76.

But what if you're already past the average life expectancy? You need to realize that life expectancy is calculated from the time of birth. An American woman who has reached age 80 actually, on average, can expect another nine years. A man at age 80 in the United States can expect almost another eight years of life, on average. And at the age of 90, women live, on average, another five years and men another four years. When you reach 100 the average life expectancy is still another two and a half years. It turns out that the older you get the healthier you have been.

What that means is if you make it through the somewhat dangerous years of the 60's and 70's, your chances of living a long life are very good. It's during the 60's and 70's when things like heart disease and cancer claim a lot of Americans.

Seven out of every ten Americans die from either cardiovascular disease (heart attack or stroke) or cancer. If you're going to have a long, healthy life you need to beat those two.

More than 1 million heart attacks occur every year

in the United States. That's one every 90 seconds. It's your number one health threat. One third of heart attack victims die within days or months of their heart attack.

What's worse is that the most common *first* symptom that you have heart disease is that you die. That's the most common first symptom. That doesn't leave you many options. You need to find out what's going on in your body *before* you have that first symptom.

GO TO WWW.THEHEALTHYLIFESUMMIT.COM TO LEARN ABOUT MY MOST ADVANCED PROGRAM OFFERING.

By the way, smokers are 2½ times more likely to get heart disease than non-smokers. More than eighty percent of people with diabetes die from some form of heart or blood vessel disease. Unfortunately, a third of the diabetics living in the United States don't even know they have diabetes.

Cancer claims over a half-million people every year in the US. The four big cancer killers are lung cancer, colon cancer, breast cancer, and prostate cancer. Half of those deaths are preventable.

In Parts 3 and 4, we'll look at what you can do to defeat the two big killers. But first, let's meet a group who are already successfully practicing The Longevity Recipe.

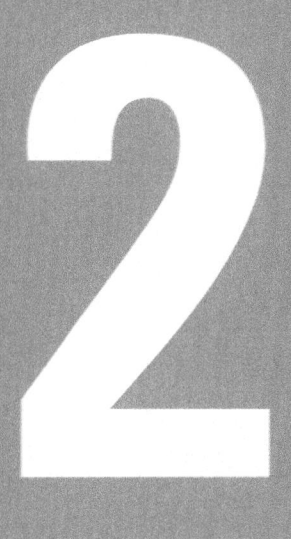

PART 2: CHAMPIONS OF LONGEVITY

2
CHAMPIONS OF LONGEVITY

LONG-LIVED AMERICANS

While lots of attention has been focused on long-lived populations in other parts of the world, here in the United States we have our own longevity champions. The Seventh-Day Adventists are a worldwide Christian denomination of 18 million members that worships on Saturday rather than Sunday. They currently have the greatest longevity of any group in America. Seventh-Day Adventist men can live as much as 11 years longer than their American counterparts. Women get a longevity boost as well.

This good health doesn't come from genetics. The Adventists are a world-wide genetically diverse group. They have good health because they practice good health habits.

The Seventh-Day Adventist faith discourages smoking, alcohol consumption, and eating the unclean foods identified in the Bible such as pork and shellfish. The Seventh-Day Adventists' strong religious beliefs have given them that extra incentive needed for turning good advice into actual healthy habits. Their religion encourages eating a vegetarian diet; some also avoid caffeinated beverages. But not everyone follows that advice.

> **NON-VEGETARIAN ADVENTISTS HAVE ABOUT TWICE THE RISK OF HEART DISEASE AS VEGETARIAN ADVENTISTS...**

And non-vegetarian Adventists have about an 85 percent increased risk of colon cancer compared to those Adventists that are vegetarian.

Scientists have been following the health experiences of Adventists for decades. The first study conducted between 1976 and 1988 looked at 34,000 Adventists in California and established a direct connection between lifestyle, disease, and longevity. The most recent, ongoing research includes 96,000 US and Canadian Adventists and preliminary results show that the closer the diet is to vegetarian the lower the levels of cholesterol, diabetes, high blood pressure, and metabolic syndrome. A decreased risk for colon polyps, a precursor of colon cancer, was found the higher the consumption of cooked green vegetables, brown rice, beans, and dried fruit. Those vegetarians who also ate fish at least once a month were found to have the lowest risk of colorectal cancer, even lower than pure vegans. A true vegan diet, based only on plant foods and not including any dairy or egg products, was also associated with lower body weight. For example, 55-year-old male and female vegans weighed approximately 30 pounds less then their non-vegetarian counterparts. Preliminary results also are suggesting that men who drink soy milk every day have about a 30 percent decreased risk of prostate cancer. Earlier research found beef intake in men directly related to an increased risk of fatal heart disease. Newer data is also suggesting that those meat-eating Adventists also double their risk of bladder cancer compared to vegetarian Adventists.

Researchers studying this group found that men who drank five or six glasses of water a day had a 60-70 percent less risk of fatal heart attack compared to those men who drank considerably less water. The difference in women was not as great. Drinking non-water fluids like soft drinks and coffee seemed to actually increase the risk of heart attack. They also found that those Adventists who consumed nuts at least five times a week had about half the risk of heart disease compared to those who did not.

The Adventists seem to handle stress better than most Americans by observing a sabbath day of rest. For them, the Sabbath day is something to look forward to. They don't work, they spend time with their families, they go on hikes, and they enjoy and appreciate God's creation. The Sabbath helps give them a sense of peace that contributes to their health. It's a guilt-free time when they're not officially obligated to do anything. It reminds them that they are part of the creation, not the creator. It reminds them that they don't have to have all the answers. The Sabbath reminds them that the world doesn't necessarily revolve around them. It helps keep their lives in perspective. It sounds like a real good idea to me.

By the way, the historic Battle Creek health sanitarium in Battle Creek, Michigan was started way back in 1876 as a Seventh-Day Adventist institution. It could accommodate more than 600 patients at a time and its first medical professional was a man by the name of John Harvey Kellogg. Kellogg and his brother, WK Kellogg, accidentally discovered the process for making flaked cereal when they were looking for an alternative to the standard "biscuits, gravy and bacon and egg breakfast" of the day. Dr. Kellogg was also the inventor of the mechanical horse and the first-generation of exercise equipment. One of Kellogg's patients was Charles W. Post who went on to introduce Post *Toasties* corn flakes and later invented *Grape Nuts* as an alternative to corn flakes. Post *Sugar Smacks* and Kellogg's *Sugar Frosted Flakes* came much later.

Here are some other conclusions from the Adventist studies.

BECOMING A VEGETARIAN WILL ADD ABOUT TWO YEARS TO YOUR LIFE SPAN.

Eating nuts on a regular basis also increases longevity by about two years. Physical activity will add several extra years as well. Interestingly, most of the benefit came from modest, but regular physical activity; marathon runners did not get a longevity boost. Maintaining a normal body weight seems to be important, too. Those Seventh-Day Adventists who ate a vegetarian diet, never smoked, maintained a healthy weight, got exercise, and ate nuts five times a week, lived 10 years longer than those Adventists who did none of those things. That's a pretty good longevity list right there! And these people are not only living longer lives, but better lives. Throughout their extended lifetimes, both physical and mental health are measured and at virtually every age the Adventists are doing better than the average American. Fortunately, you don't have to do everything they do to get some benefit. The bottom line is that even modest changes to the average American's current lifestyle can help a lot.

PART 2: CHAMPIONS OF LONGEVITY

PART 3

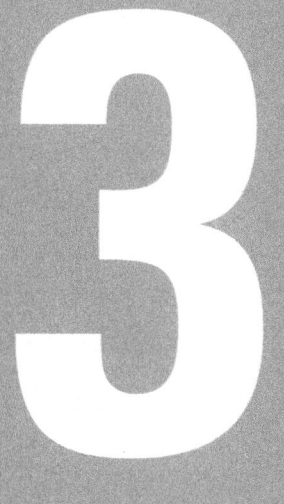

BEAT HEART DISEASE

DON'T TRUST YOUR CHOLESTEROL NUMBER

You already know that you need to watch your cholesterol. But does that mean you need to watch how much cholesterol you eat or watch your blood cholesterol number? Or both?

Science has known for sometime that, for the average person, the amount of cholesterol you eat, like in an egg yolk, does NOT make your blood cholesterol number go up very much. What does make it go up is the amount of saturated fat that you consume. Saturated fat and dietary cholesterol are two different things. Only one of them significantly affects your blood cholesterol numbers.

THE MOST RECENT GUIDELINES SUGGEST LIMITING TOTAL SATURATED FAT INTAKE TO ABOUT 13 GRAMS PER DAY. THAT MEANS LOOKING AT THE LABELS OF WHAT YOU BUY AND EATING LESS ANIMAL PRODUCTS.

Recently, a major study said that decreasing saturated fat did NOT improve your cardiovascular health. *The New York Times* even ran a headline that said "Butter Is Back." They sold a lot of newspapers that day. However, the media is usually interested in headlines, not in the details. What wasn't pointed out is the fact that decreasing saturated fat in your diet DOES decrease your cardiovascular risk IF you replace it with oils like omega-3's and olive oil. On the other hand, if saturated fats are replaced with sugar and processed foods, then no benefit is seen. The devil, as usual, is in the details. Yes, do eat less animal and saturated fats.

And beware, a finger prick that only gives you

PART 3: BEAT HEART DISEASE

your total blood cholesterol number doesn't tell you much, especially since we now have so many more advanced blood tests. A blood cholesterol value of under 200 may have been reassuring during the 1980's, but not anymore. You need more information than that. At the very least, get your total cholesterol, HDL, LDL, triglycerides, LP(a), and Lp-PLA2 levels measured. Be sure to get retested regularly. If your numbers don't start improving after six months of better health habits, ask your physician about medication. High cholesterol numbers are serious! Don't wait for something to go wrong. Remember, they call it the silent killer for a reason. Prevent a heart attack before it happens!

We now know that there are a lot more factors that can affect your heart disease risk. It turns out that having a healthy lifestyle, getting a flu shot, taking a baby aspirin, losing a couple pounds off your mid-section, and finding out if you have insulin resistance all can have a profound impact on protecting you from America's big killer. Let's look at the specifics.

LIVE THE GOOD LIFE

Living a healthy lifestyle is still the single most effective way to decrease your personal risk of cardiovascular disease. It beats out drugs and surgery by far. A Canadian study that interviewed 32,000 people from forty countries found that even those that already had cardiovascular disease were still less likely to die from it or have another heart attack or stroke if they ate a healthy diet. Unfortunately, for some people, especially those that have inherited poor genetics, myself included, lifestyle is often not enough. It must be the foundation, but in many cases it needs to be complemented with medicines.

Your number one dietary goal is to eat less animal fat, also known as saturated fat. Among the top sources are pizza, cheese, meat, and whole dairy products. Over time, replace those fats with better choices like olive oil, the omega-3's in fish, and the fats found in nuts. Eat more fruits, vegetables, and whole grain products, as well. Research shows that if you'll stick with a healthier diet for six months, your taste buds will start to cooper-

PART 3: BEAT HEART DISEASE

ate with you. You'll begin to like your new way of eating.

If you've been told to decrease your salt intake, you'll need to start using the salt shaker again. That's correct. Surprisingly, 75 percent of the salt we eat in this country comes from processed foods, not the salt shaker. So, put the salt shaker back on the table and use it with lower-salt or no-salt versions of your favorite foods. That way, you really can lower your salt intake and still eat food that tastes good.

And be sure to put some physical activity into your lifestyle. Even if you already have heart disease, physical activity can help your body's blood vessels build collateral circulation around narrowed arteries. As a result, even if an artery becomes blocked, there may still be enough blood flow to your heart muscle to prevent what otherwise might be a full-blown heart attack or even death. That physical activity may help you lose some weight and get your blood pressure under control, too. Simply losing excess body fat will bring the blood pressure of many adults back to normal. If you're on medication now, you may need to decrease the dosage after you lose weight. Work with your physician.

And of course, stop smoking now! Use a patch,

chew the gum, take the pill, do whatever it takes. The very best thing you can do for your heart and your health is to get tobacco products out of your life!

TAKE A SHOT

Every year 91,000 Americans die from a heart attack or stroke triggered by the flu. A large study found that when those with cardiovascular disease get a flu shot they cut their risk of having another cardiovascular event by 50 percent. Fifty percent! And as if that isn't enough, you decrease your chances of getting the flu! Remember the last time you had the flu? Remember how miserable you were? Remember the last time you had a heart attack? Remember how you almost died? Go to Walgreens and get a flu shot. No appointment necessary.

Have your doctor give you a shingles shot, too. Everyone over 60 should get one and those over 50 with cardiovascular disease should get one as well. The shot reduces the risk of shingles by about 70 percent. If you've ever known anyone with shingles, and see the agony they go through, you WILL get the shot. Besides, people who get shingles are up to four times as likely to have a stroke. If you ever had chickenpox, you need to get the shingles vaccine. If you are over 65 you need to get a pneumonia shot as well. If you have cardiovascular disease, and are 50 or over, you need to get one, too. Regardless of your age, if you get a pneumonia shot your risk of having a heart attack or stroke goes down. So get a flu shot, get a shingles shot, and one to help prevent pneumonia as well. Just go do it. Yes, I know that's a lot of shots. But if you're going to die from something, die from something we don't know how to cure. Don't let your life get cut short from something we already know how to prevent or fix. That would just be dumb.

ACT LIKE A BABY

Aspirin helps prevent a heart attack or stroke by decreasing your blood platelets ability to stick together and form clots. That's the normal function of platelets. But if plaque in your arteries ruptures, your body will attempt to fix the rupture by forming a blood clot around it. If that clot gets big enough, it will impede blood flow in that particular artery and cause a heart attack or stroke. A low dose (baby) aspirin of 81 mg a day specifically targets something called the COX–1 enzyme that makes platelets stick together. Full strength aspirin at 325 mg works on both COX–1 and COX–2 enzymes. By blocking the COX–2 enzyme, aspirin gets its well-deserved reputation as being a pain and fever reliever. But the COX–2 enzyme also beneficially widens arteries and fights blood clots. So, we don't want to inhibit the COX–2 enzyme with a full strength aspirin. Frequent use of Ibuprofen (Advil and Motrin), which also inhibits the COX-2 enzyme, has also been found to nearly triple the risk of stroke for similar reasons.

A simple, inexpensive genetic test is now available to see how you personally respond to aspirin therapy. About 30 percent of the US has some degree of aspirin resistance. Those that have this genetic resistance and have current arterial disease are up to four times more likely to suffer some kind of cardiovascular event. It's good to know if you're one of those people. Additionally, it's good to know if you're taking aspirin whether or not your body is responding appropriately. If you have aspirin resistance one baby aspirin may not be giving you the benefit you expect. If you are aspirin resistant, your physician may choose to increase your baby aspirin dose to two per day. You won't know unless you take the test. Ask your physician about the "Aspirin Resistance Test."

SUCK IT IN

Assuming you don't smoke, your number one health priority is to slowly take excess weight off your body. The best way to do that is to eat less fat and sugar and put physical activity into your lifestyle. But we now understand that it's not just how much you weigh, but where you carry your weight that matters. Especially where you carry your extra weight. When you go to a doctor's office, they usually put you on the scale. If they don't get a tape measure out, and measure your waist size, you may want to find another physician. We know that belly fat is metabolically very active tissue. The fat stored in your midsection easily goes in and out of your blood circulation. That can contribute to all kinds of health problems.

If you're a woman, you may have noticed that the

man in your life has a much easier time of losing weight than you do. Why is that? It's because when he needs calories for exercise they are readily released from where he has a lot stored; his belly. But where do women store a lot of their body fat? On the hips. Unfortunately, once fat ends up on your hips, it likes it back there! The fat stored on your hips is not very metabolically active. You know that because of how hard it is to get rid of it. It's easier to lose belly fat than to lose hip fat. Now, granted, this isn't fair. But you're probably old enough to know life isn't fair.

While it may be easier to lose gut fat than hip fat, this mid-section fat is also contributing to an increased cholesterol level, higher triglyceride levels, and all kinds of other increased risk factors in his life. Not good things. That's why twenty extra pounds on a man is more dangerous than twenty extra pounds on a woman; because of where it's stored.

As a result of this, we can use a tape measure to help predict your future. As we said earlier, to keep this risk factor under control, we know that a man's waist size should not go above 40 inches. For a woman, it shouldn't go above 35 inches. That's true for whites, blacks, and Hispanics. For Asians, men's waist sizes should not go above 35 inches; for Asian women, 31 inches.

Where you measure is not necessarily where you would think. It's not at the bellybutton level. If you press on your lower abdomen you should be able to find two protruding bones at the top of your pelvis. This is called the iliac crest. Now if you can't find those bones… that's a risk factor right there! Measuring at the iliac crest level, parallel to the floor, go all the way around your body to get your official waist measurement. If you're above the target cutoff for waist size, you're at an increased risk for all kinds of future health problems including something called "insulin resistance."

DON'T RESIST

The disease you just might have, that you haven't even heard about, is insulin resistance. First, a basic review. Insulin is the substance secreted by your pancreas that allows blood sugar into your cells. Without insulin, the food you eat cannot get into the cells to be metabolized. About 1 in 3 adults have insulin resistance and 90 percent of them don't know it. Unless they do something about it, about 70 percent of those with insulin resistance will go on to become diabetic in their lifetime. In insulin resistance, the cells don't respond as well to the insulin as they should. As a result, the blood sugar stays high. This high circulating sugar makes your arteries more susceptible to damage. As a result, insulin resistance also increases risk for coronary artery disease. Your risk for damage to the kidneys, eyes, and nerves also goes up with insulin resistance. The risk for dementia increases as well.

> **UNFORTUNATELY, YOU CAN HAVE NORMAL BLOOD SUGAR LEVELS AND STILL HAVE INSULIN RESISTANCE.**

The pancreas can simply pump out more and more insulin so that eventually the blood sugar can enter the cell, even though it is resistant to a normal amount of insulin. It can do that for years and years and a standard blood sugar test or even an A1C will show normal levels. But eventually, the beta-cells of the pancreas can't make enough insulin and that's when the blood sugar stays high and a diagnosis of diabetes is made.

Most physicians today are not testing for insulin resistance. The test, called an oral glucose tolerance test (OGTT), follows what happens to your blood sugar levels for two hours after taking a high challenge dose of 75 grams of glucose after an overnight fast. Fasting blood sugar and A1C are not as dependable as the OGTT. You need to get this test done. If you have insulin resistance, it's contributing to your cardiovascular disease risk and you need to take steps to get it under control. Exercise, losing weight, and cutting down on soda and all sweetened beverages will help. Research also suggests that emphasizing foods rich in magnesium like leafy greens, whole grains, nuts, and beans, can decrease insulin resistance too. A magnesium supplement of somewhere between 300-400mg per day may also help.

Research shows that if you have insulin resistance you can decrease your chances of going on to diabetes by about 60 percent if you will exercise about 30 minutes a day, 5 days a week and lose just 7 percent of your body weight. If you're overweight at 200 pounds, that means losing 14 pounds. You do NOT have to get to your ideal body weight to see health benefits.

YOU'RE JUST GETTING STARTED

Frankly, we've just scratched the surface here. There is SO much more you need to know to beat the biggest killer. You can get my book *The Enemy Within* at my website www.DavidMeinz.com and for more detailed, potentially life-saving information go to: www.TheHealthyLifeSummit.com There you'll find the latest information on my most advanced program offering, and some informative video, too. You'll learn a lot.

PART 3: BEAT HEART DISEASE

PART 4: PREVENT CANCER

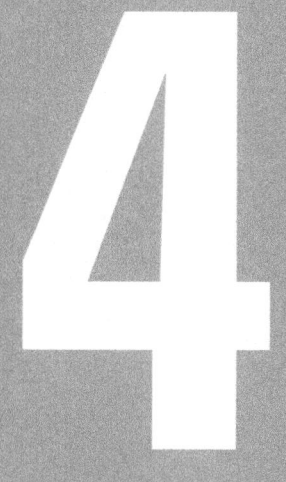

4
PREVENT CANCER

OVER A HALF MILLION A YEAR

Fifteen hundred people died today from cancer. About 1,000 of them didn't have to. We already know enough to prevent two-thirds of all cancers. What we don't know yet is how to get people to take responsibility for their own health.

As deadly as heart disease is, many people fear a diagnosis of cancer even more. When I worked at a hospital I'd hear physicians and nurses talking about "C-A." It took me a while to figure out they were discussing patients with CAncer. Even some health professionals are uncomfortable saying the word. The fear is justified.

Cancer causes one out of every four deaths in this country and is the second biggest killer. Cancer causes pain that can linger for months and even years.

Many people mistakenly believe that heart disease is a rather quick way to go. But, in fact, today many people who have a heart attack survive. More often than not, though, they never return to the same quality of life they had before their heart attack. Additionally, the same dangerous process that often brings on quick heart attacks also causes strokes, and the effects of a stroke can last the rest of your lifetime. Neither cancer nor heart disease is a good way to go, and neither is better than the other.

Of the half-million-plus people in the United States who die each year from cancer, most of them could still be alive and well if they had stopped smoking and improved the quality of the food they ate.

Get cigarettes and all tobacco products out of your life. Get help. Your addiction to nicotine is no stronger than it was for the millions and millions of people who are now successful former smokers. Whatever it takes, see to it that the young people in your life never start smoking or using tobacco products. A lifetime of good health is among the best legacies you'll ever leave for your children and grandchildren.

Everyone knows smoking causes cancer. Most people still don't know that a poor diet causes about the same number of cancer cases. The bottom line on nutrition and cancer prevention is to increase fruits and vegetables and to decrease saturated fat and red and processed meats. Taking excess body fat off will help as well.

GOOD NUTRITION CAN HELP REDUCE YOUR OVERALL CANCER RISK TOO.

Eating more foods rich in beta-carotene like cantaloupe, carrots, sweet potatoes, broccoli, and spinach will help. Vitamin C foods are also effective and include citrus fruits, strawberries, and tomatoes.

Avoiding or really cutting back on alcohol consumption and limiting your intake of salt-cured, smoked, and nitrite-cured foods are also good ideas.

There's an old proverb that says, "Put a knife to your throat if you are given to gluttony." There's evidence now that a high-calorie diet also significantly increases a person's risk for colon cancer. Obesity in your midsection seems to be risky as well. We know from lab studies that if you restrict calories in those animals that already have cancer, you can prevent the tumors from growing and can stop new ones from developing. Cancer cells, like all cells, need energy to grow. With excessively high calorie intake, you may simply be stoking the fire of cancer growth.

SLOW BUT STEADY PROGRESS IS BEING MADE ON THOSE CANCERS THAT AREN'T DIRECTLY RELATED TO LIFESTYLE.

In the 1930s, the average cancer patient had only a 20 percent chance of being alive in five years. In the 1940s it was up to 25 percent, and by the 1960s it was 30 percent. Today the average five-year survival rate is 40 percent.

You may not be impressed with that kind of progress if you're the one with cancer, but the news is far better than it appears. The average five-year survival rate is so modest because it includes lung cancer. If you exclude that particular disease, the rate is much better.

In the last 30 years, deaths from colorectal cancer are down 9 percent in men and down 31 percent in women. Liver cancer deaths are down 13 percent in men and down 45 percent in women, and deaths from stomach cancer are down about 60 percent in both men and women. Bladder cancer and Hodgkin's disease are also both down, and the cancer death rate in children is down a reassuring 62 percent!

Early detection before the cancer spreads has a lot to do with your chance of beating this killer. The American Cancer Society recommends that women be sure to do regular breast self-exams and, after age 45, get annual mammograms. On the other hand, the U.S. Preventive Services Task Force says a woman can wait till age 50 for a mammography every other year. If you're a man over 40, have your doctor check your prostate as part of your regular medical checkups. Many health experts recommend that men over age 50 should also have the PSA blood test done as well, although the American Academy of Family Physicians advises against routine PSA testing. And if you're a man or woman over 50, get tested for colon and rectal cancer. Better to go through a little discomfort now than experience the pain of surgery—or worse—later. Your odds of preventing cancer are far, far greater than your chances of getting cured from it.

The *2015 Estimated US Cancer Deaths* and *Trends in Age-Related Cancer Deaths* tables (pages 129-131) clearly show that the main cancer threats to women are lung, breast, and colorectal cancers. For men the cancer threats are lung, prostate, and colorectal. Breast cancer gets so much publicity when, in fact, lung cancer kills far more women every year. Perhaps in addition to encouraging women to get regular mammograms, we should put even more effort into keeping their teenage daughters from lighting up their first cigarette. If current trends continue, the incredible number of new teenage female smokers will become the future victims of lung cancer as adults.

While many adults will someday be told they have cancer, it's no longer a death sentence. The very good news is that more people are beating cancer than ever before.

No technology or medicine can make you stop smoking. The decision must come from within you. No device or drug will lift you off the couch or make you eat broccoli. The desire to live long enough to see your grandchildren grow up—and the effort to do something about it—must come from you alone. Regardless of any new breakthroughs in cancer research, the information already known can help most of us beat cancer before it ever starts.

2015 ESTIMATED US CANCER DEATHS

LEADING CANCER DEATHS IN FEMALES

Lung & bronchus	71,660
Breast	40,290
Colon & rectum	23,600
Pancreas	19,850
Ovary	14,180
Leukemia	10,240
Uterine corpus	10,170
Non-Hodgkin lymphoma	8,310
Liver & intrahepatic bile duct	7,520
Brain & other nervous system	6,360

LEADING CANCER DEATHS IN MALES

Lung & bronchus	86,380
Prostate	27,540
Colon & rectum	26,100
Pancreas	20,710
Liver & intrahepatic bile duct	17,030
Leukemia	14,210
Esophagus	12,600
Urinary bladder	11,510
Non-Hodgkin lymphoma	11,480
Kidney & renal pelvis	9,070

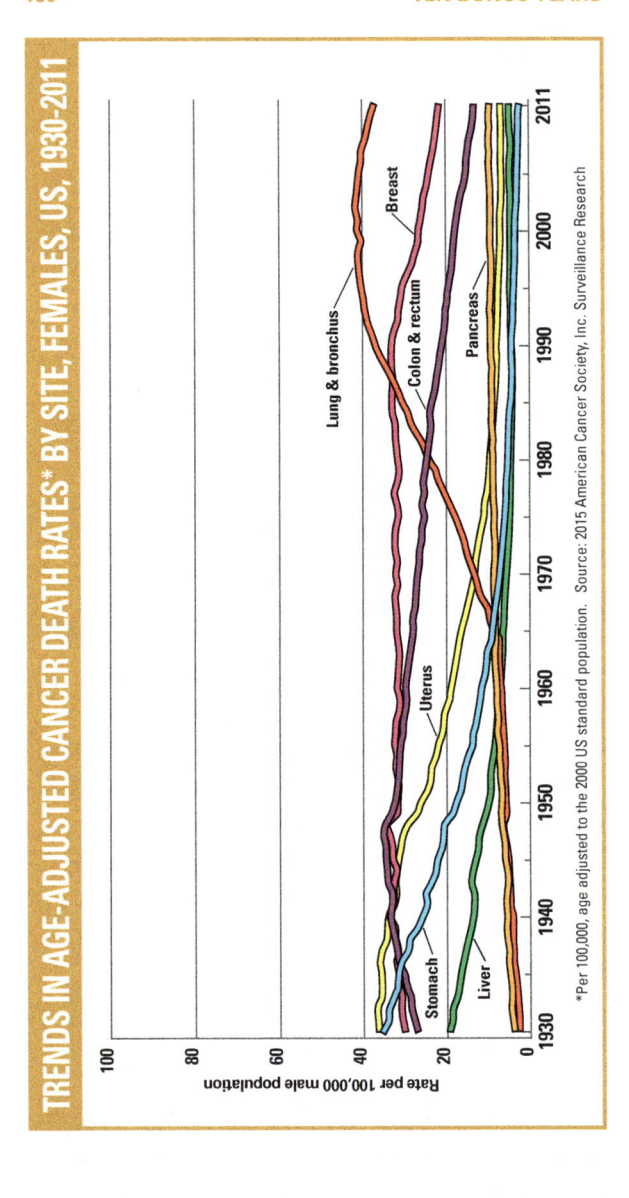

TRENDS IN AGE-ADJUSTED CANCER DEATH RATES* BY SITE, FEMALES, US, 1930–2011

*Per 100,000, age adjusted to the 2000 US standard population. Source: 2015 American Cancer Society, Inc. Surveillance Research

PART 4: PREVENT CANCER 131

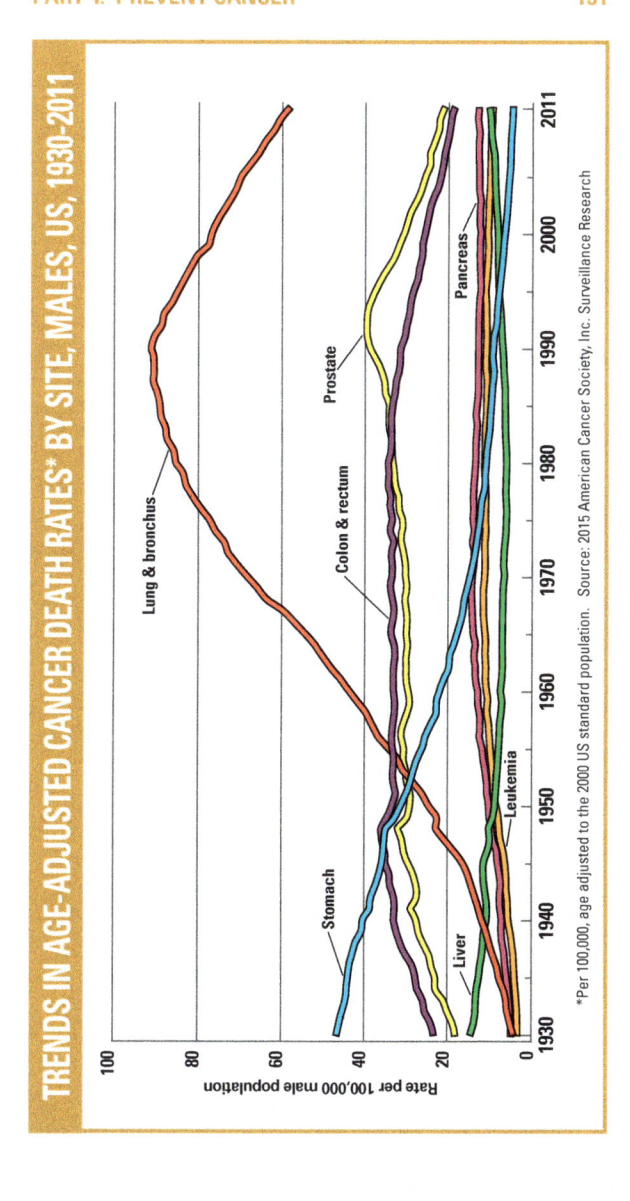

TRENDS IN AGE-ADJUSTED CANCER DEATH RATES* BY SITE, MALES, US, 1930-2011

*Per 100,000, age adjusted to the 2000 US standard population. Source: 2015 American Cancer Society, Inc. Surveillance Research

# PART 5: EAT LIKE AN ITALIAN

5
EAT LIKE AN ITALIAN

LET'S MEET IN THE MIDDLE

So here's the problem. You'd like those 10 bonus years but you don't want to become a vegetarian. Tofu just doesn't do that much for you. You consider ketchup a vegetable. The good news is that you don't necessarily have to eat like an Adventist, just as long as you don't eat like an American. A healthy middle ground may be to eat more like an Italian. Over the last several years more and more research is pointing to the benefits of eating what's called "The Mediterranean Diet." This approach is based on the dietary habits of people living on the island of Crete, off the coast of Italy, as well as on the diets of the people in southern Italy and the rest of Greece in the early part of the 1950's. Back in 1952 Dr. Ancel Keys from the University of Minnesota started research on the health experience and diets of seven different countries around the world. They included Yugoslavia, Italy, Greece, The Netherlands, Finland, the United States, and Japan. Even though it's common knowledge today, he was the first one to discover that people who had a diet high in saturated fats also had high blood cholesterol levels and the greatest incidence of heart attack. He found that the highest risk of heart disease was in Finland where they also had the highest intake of dietary fat. He reported people slicing large slabs of cheese and putting butter on it for a snack.(!) He found that the lowest fat intake was in Japan, where a lot of rice and fish was, and still is, consumed. What's surprising, however, was that the people in Japan did not have the lowest rate of heart disease. In fact, it was the Italians that had the best health outcomes, even though they weren't eating the lowest amount of fat.

In fact, the Mediterranean diet back then usually got somewhere between thirty and forty percent of its calories from fat. That's higher than has been traditionally recommended in the US. What's important is that they did not have a high animal fat intake and that, apparently, is the key. The diet of these very healthy Italians is interesting to observe. It included a lot of olive oil and whole grain bread. They also ate beans, fresh fruit and vegetables, and a lot of dark leafy greens; foods like Swiss chard, kale, spinach, and mustard greens sautéed in a little olive oil or garlic. Sugar and most dairy foods were very rare. Of the dairy they did eat, it was usually yogurt and some cheese used as a condiment, not in large quantities. They also ate a little fish and chicken a couple times a week. Red meat was only consumed several times a month.

IT'S GOOD AND GOOD FOR YOU

It turns out that the Mediterranean diet is good for your heart. Researchers in Greece followed 22,000 people for four years and found that those eating the traditional Greek diet were 33 percent less likely to die from heart disease than Greeks eating other foods. If you've already had a heart attack, eating this way appears to greatly reduce your risk of having a second one. What's more, another study showed that after just three months those on a traditional Mediterranean diet with olive oil had a decrease in levels of the dangerous oxidized LDL in the blood and blood pressure went down as well. And it's never too late to get benefit from this way of eating. A study that looked at 2,300 people aged 70 to 90 found that those following the Mediterranean diet had a 23 percent decrease in death rate from heart disease, cancer, and stroke.

> **THOSE THAT ALSO EXERCISED, KEPT THEIR ALCOHOL AT MODERATE LEVELS, AND DIDN'T SMOKE, HAD A 65 PERCENT LOWER DEATH RATE!**

A study reported in the *Journal of The American Medical Association* found that the diet can also help those with metabolic syndrome. That's a problem shared by about 25 percent of all Americans and is a combination of obesity and large waist size, high blood pressure, low levels of the good HDL cholesterol, and increased blood sugar. That particular combination of risk factors dramatically increases your risk of cardiovascular disease. The researchers found that those people with metabolic syndrome that followed the Mediterranean diet for two years lost weight; decreased insulin resistance and inflammation; lowered their blood sugar, cholesterol, and triglyceride levels;

PART 5: EAT LIKE AN ITALIAN

and had lower blood pressure when compared to those people who were put on just a low fat, low cholesterol diet. What's more, those on the Mediterranean diet increased their good HDL cholesterol levels and a full half of them no longer had metabolic syndrome. That's better than any medicine can accomplish. All they did was cut down on their animal fat and eat more fruits, vegetables, beans, nuts, whole grains, olive oil, and the healthy omega-3 fats from fish. That doesn't sound too bad, does it?

The Mediterranean diet also appears to reduce your risk of getting certain cancers as well. In one large Italian study it was found that vegetable consumption decreased risk of cancers of the upper respiratory and digestive track. In a different four-year study, looking at about 600 men and women, researchers found that those who were eating the Mediterranean type diet were about 60 percent less likely to develop cancers in the following years compared to those who ate the often recommended reduced fat and cholesterol diet. A study that followed 22,000 Greeks for four years found that those eating the traditional diet were 24 percent less likely to die from cancer.

You may be able to help keep your mind sharp from eating like an Italian, too. The *Journal of The*

American Medical Association recently published the results of a long-term study of 447 individuals. They were assigned to a Mediterranean-style diet with either 30 grams of walnuts, almonds, or hazelnuts every day or one liter of extra virgin olive oil per week, or to the control group who were advised to eat a low-fat diet. At the average follow-up of about four years, subjects were tested on cognitive functions such as memory and attention span. Both groups assigned to the Mediterranean diets had improved over-all cognition, while the low-fat diet group had a decrease in mental function.

If you eat like an Italian you may have less to worry about when it comes to Alzheimer's disease, as well. A study looking at over 2200 elderly for four years found that those that ate closest to a Mediterranean diet decreased their risk of developing Alzheimer's by about 40 percent. The researchers said that the high quality of vitamins and nutrients in this diet may help decrease inflammation and oxidation in the body. Since we already know that brain health is related to cardiovascular health it just may be that since the Mediterranean diet is good for your heart it may also be doing your brain some good, too.

Want more good news? It looks like the Mediterranean diet may also decrease your chances of getting diabetes, too. Researchers in Spain tracked the health of some 13,000 men and women for four years. They found that those who followed this way of eating were 83 percent less likely to develop type-2 diabetes.

HERE'S WHAT YOU SHOULD EAT

So what goes into a good Mediterranean diet, especially as it was consumed in the 1950's? Breads, cereals, pastas, and grain products are a staple that's included in every meal. But unlike many American diets, we're talking whole grain products here such as whole wheat bread and pasta. Relax, you're NOT going to get fat on the carbohydrates in the Mediterranean diet. As far as protein is concerned, the Mediterranean diet depends largely on legumes, peas, beans and lentils. Like whole grain products, beans are also loaded with fiber. Fish is another great source of protein and it's usually consumed several times a week. Of course, fish provides the good heart healthy omega-3 fats which help keep the blood flowing and decreases the risk for a heart attack. Nuts including almonds, hazel nuts, and pistachios are also regularly consumed.

You hardly ever see a piece of pie or cake in the Mediterranean diet. Cakes and high sugar desserts are reserved for special occasions, but they rarely are a part of the traditional meal. Every meal does seem to finish with some kind of sweet, but it's fruit. Just simple, whole fruit. Among the favorites are oranges, apricots, pears, apples, figs, and peaches. You can't go wrong with fruits and vegetables and this is an area where Americans fall short. Fortunately, the Mediterranean diet does include things that a lot of us already enjoy such as tomatoes, zucchini, onions, carrots, broccoli, and peppers. The research is indicating that vegetables and fruits, beyond their obvious benefits of vitamins and minerals, are a powerhouse of those phytochemicals and antioxidants that seem to play a role in decreasing your risk for cancer. In addition to the healthy substances found in the red wine that's consumed, some research suggests that the vitamin E found in traditional Mediterranean food has an equally protective effect against coronary artery disease.

NOT POPEYE'S GIRLFRIEND

Unlike many countries around the world, the primary source of fat in the Mediterranean diet is olive oil. Mediterraneans and Italians use it everywhere and in everything. They don't spread saturated butter fat on their bread, they sprinkle olive oil on it. They put it in salads, they sauté in it, and they use it in cooking vegetables.

The research is still unclear, however, on whether olive oil itself, specifically what we call a monounsaturated fat, is a key component of the good health outcomes of the Mediterranean way of eating. Of course, you're always better off eating any unsaturated fat compared to a saturated animal fat. To be on the safe side though, you can't go wrong with a monounsaturated fat like canola or olive oil.

We Americans are still getting somewhere between 35 and 38 percent of our daily calories from fat. Interestingly, the original research done back in the 1950's observed that people in Greece were eating as much as 40 percent of their calories from fat. That's a huge amount.

Since it was primarily olive oil, heart disease risk wasn't increased. However, obesity might have been expected since "fat is fat is fat" when it comes to calories. The reason that these people were able to consume so much fat in those days without weight gain was primarily because they were mostly farmers; they burned a huge amount of calories every day in heavy manual labor.

OLIVE OIL CERTAINLY SEEMS TO BE HEALTHFUL, BUT DON'T START FRYING EVERYTHING IN OLIVE OIL!

What's the difference between extra virgin, virgin, regular, and light olive oil? Olive oil is categorized by its flavor, aroma, color and its acidity level. Extra virgin olive oil has an absolutely perfect taste, aroma, and a fruity flavor. There are subtle flavor differences in extra virgin olive oil based on the climate where the olives are raised and the makeup of the soil. Extra virgin olive oil has the strongest most definite olive taste and, by definition, it can have an acidity level of no more than one percent. It's best used in salads and on breads as a topping. Virgin olive oil, on the other hand, is produced the same way as extra virgin is, but it's acidity level can be anywhere between one and three percent. That doesn't mean much to the consumer, but it is an industry standard. Finally, just plain olive oil is that which has some kind of an off taste or acidity level greater than three percent and it's not really considered acceptable for human consumption. So, they process and refine it and then it's combined with virgin olive oil to get what you see in the store labeled simply as "olive oil." If you're using oil with something that requires it to be heated, you can probably just use this cheaper regular olive oil since it loses some of its flavor upon heating anyway. Today, you can also buy "extra light" olive oil. This is just plain olive oil that's lighter in color. There's no strong flavor and a lot of people prefer this variety. But be careful, just because it says "extra light" doesn't mean it's lower in fat or calories; it's exactly the same as all other olive oils. It's just that a lot of people prefer the lighter taste.

Another question that often comes up regarding oils are the terms "first pressing" and "cold pressed" oil. These terms really don't mean anything any more. First pressing indicated oil that indeed came out of the first pressing of the olive and then the olive was subjected to other pressings down the line. All oil now is first pressed. Cold pressed oil is not important any more either since almost all oil is now cold pressed; heat is no longer used during the extraction of the oil from the olive.

What does this all mean to you? Of the oil that you do use, I recommend that you try to go with olive oil or, as we said earlier, canola oil. You can use olive oil in any place where you would be using regular vegetable oil. Just find one whose taste you like. If you're making light or delicate dishes like fish, chicken, or veal, you might want to go with the milder regular olive oil or "extra light." If you're making stews, heartier flavored dishes, tomato based sauces, as well as steamed vegetables and salads, then extra virgin is a good choice.

By the way, olive oil isn't the only oil that's good for your heart. Replacing saturated animal fats in your diet with any unsaturated fat, like olive, canola, soy, or vegetable oil is also healthful. It's just that olive oil is the unsaturated oil of choice in the very healthy Mediterranean diet. Of course, you can always get too much of a good thing. When you see that little bowl of olive oil on the table next time you're at an Italian restaurant, just remember it's got 120 calories in a tablespoon, the same as any other oil. So go easy on dipping that bread.

And a word about olives themselves. Initially you might think they're off limits since they get between 75-85 percent of their calories from fat. But that's only because olives have so few total calories to begin with. Obviously, if a food doesn't have many calories, any fat that it does have is going to make a larger percentage contribution. In fact, a typical half-ounce serving of black or green olives only has 1½ grams of fat. Here's an example of why I don't like to teach percentages, but actual grams of something in a serving. If you went just by the fat percentage of olives you wouldn't eat them. But when you realize how really low in fat they are you see that they're just fine.

In addition to olive oil, every good italian dish contains at least a little garlic. Recent research on this pungent bulb has been surprising.

CONTRARY TO EARLIER STUDIES THAT INDICATED THAT GARLIC WOULD REDUCE BLOOD CHOLESTEROL, THE VERY BEST RESEARCH DOES NOT BACK THAT UP.

However, garlic does seem to have an antibacterial and anti-clotting effect. Some research also suggests that it may help reduce blood pressure as well. It can also reduce the number of friends you have. So how do you eat garlic and maintain your social connections? Crush it and then bake it slightly. The substances called thiosulfinates found in both garlic and onions not only make your eyes water but they're what helps lower blood pressure and keep your blood platelets from causing dangerous clots. Experts had thought that the only way to get the benefit from these thiosulfinates was to eat the garlic or onion raw. We now know, however, that lightly boiling or baking crushed cloves of garlic gives you almost all of the same health benefits as eating it raw, without all the bad breath. Interestingly, scientists have discovered that microwaving does destroy these beneficial compounds. Stick to baking or boiling.

I'LL DRINK TO THAT?

Other than at breakfast, wine consumption is a normal part of every meal in the Mediterranean world. Average intakes are about two glasses of wine a day for a man and one glass of wine a day for a woman. But a key component of that alcohol consumption may be that it's always consumed with food. Unlike in the US, in the Mediterranean countries, wine or alcohol of any kind is rarely consumed by itself.

A study in Denmark has observed something of interest recently as well. Since Denmark entered the Common Market, heart disease death rate is down 30 percent. Also since entering the Common Market, wine prices have gone down in Denmark and wine consumption is up 30 percent. Is there something protective about wine?

Some research would indicate that it decreases the stickiness of the platelets in your arteries, and these platelets are what can lead to clot formation and ultimately a heart attack. So wine appears to make these platelets less sticky and less likely to clot. The study found that beer didn't have any protective effect and hard liquor only had a little.

But keep in mind, in women, there's a fine line between decreasing risk for heart disease and increasing risk for breast cancer. That line may be crossed after just one glass of wine a day.

So, should you go out and start drinking alcohol? The recommendation is that if you don't drink now, don't start. And of course, there's always the concern of alcoholism. New genetic testing now reveals that a much smaller percentage of us get cardiovascular protection from alcohol than previously thought. The good news is that you can still get most of the benefits from the Mediterranean diet without consuming alcohol.

THAT WAS THEN, THIS IS NOW

If you happen to take a trip overseas you'll find that the foods that are consumed there today by many people in the areas of southern Italy and Greece are not, in fact, what we've been describing here as the Mediterranean diet. More and more the diets of the Mediterranean people are looking like what we're eating in the United States. The influence of western society is felt not only in clothes and music, but in food as well. The Mediterranean diet we've been talking about here to a large degree no longer exists. It did exist in the 1950's and earlier but a lot of what you see in Italy and Greece today looks a lot more like what they eat in Scranton than in Sicily.

Evidence from dietary surveys is showing that there are rapid changes going on in the Mediterranean area today and they're usually going in the wrong direction. On the island of Crete, they've had an increase in meat, fish and cheese consumption, but their intake of bread, fruit, potatoes, and olive oil has all gone down. Availability of meat, dairy foods, and animal fats has gone up throughout the Mediterranean region since the early 1960's. Similar trends are being found in Italy as well. There's also less physical activity and, as a result, blood cholesterol, blood pressure, and obesity levels are all going higher. And as you would expect, levels of coronary heart disease, diabetes, and certain diet related cancers are going up, too.

Keep in mind that when you go to an Italian restaurant in the US what you're seeing there doesn't necessarily reflect the Mediterranean diet of sixty years ago. In Italian restaurants found in this country today, it's hard to get a pasta dish that's not loaded with meat sauce, butter, or cheese. Meat or sausage is often the primary item in many entrees here in Italian restaurants. Traditional American desserts like pies and cakes, not the simple fruits of the Mediterranean diet, are the standard in Italian restaurants here as well. Remember that white cream based pasta sauces are loaded with fat, especially the bad saturated fats. When it comes to pasta go with the red tomato based sauces. They're delicious, they have the health benefits of tomatoes, and they're low in fat.

While the dietary habits may not be as good in the Mediterranean countries as they were some sixty years ago, in general, they're still doing better than the rest of Europe and America. In addition to their diet, what other factors might be contributing to their overall health?

First of all, people in southern Italy and other parts of the Mediterranean tend to be very physically active as part of their daily routine. But you won't usually find them going to the gym for a daily workout. That concept is relatively unknown. But, they do walk to the market every day to get fresh fruits and vegetables and then they walk back home. They walk to get fresh baked bread and they walk back home. Many take a walk after dinner, too. As a matter of fact, walking by foot is often the most common mode of transportation. They work and take care of their daily routine close to where they live.

They're also much less likely to watch the incredible amounts of television that most Americans do. They drink wine in moderation with meals, but water is the other preferred beverage. Soda doesn't have much appeal.

Another characteristic of the Mediterranean culture is that they tend to have a high degree of social support. This seems to be important for long-term health and stress management. The way meals are prepared and served is also a good indication of this social support. It's rather unusual to see somebody driving through McDonalds in southern Italy to grab a quick five-minute meal. Instead, the people that are still benefiting from the traditional Mediterranean way of eating often make a meal a 2-hour affair.

> **FAMILY, FRIENDS, LAUGHTER, AND ENJOYABLE EXPERIENCES ALL NOURISH BOTH THE MIND AND THE BODY.**

In some of the cultures of the Mediterranean area they actually still practice the afternoon rest or siesta. Many of us in the good ol' USA look upon that as just plain wasted time. Yet in the healthy Mediterranean culture it may, in fact, be contributing to the health that we over here are so desperately seeking. Stress can have a significant influence on your health. A quick nap, a time talking with friends, or something that gets you out of the grind for a short amount of time, all seem to play a big role in reducing that stress.

EATING LIKE THEM, OVER HERE

So what does all this mean for you and your family? Let's look at some practical, take home suggestions that you can use. Remember, the Mediterranean diet tastes very good; this isn't some food plan you have to tolerate. When you eat like an Italian you get lots of food and you'll like how it tastes, too.

First of all, eat more vegetables; canned, fresh, frozen, just eat more vegetables. Only about 25 percent of Americans eat the recommended amount every day. Eat more tomatoes, more broccoli, more carrots, and more sweet potatoes. If you can get them fresh, like at a farmer's market, that's great. Some people think that unless produce is fresh it has no value. Not true. Contrary to popular belief, canned green beans contain almost the same nutrition as fresh and frozen. Remember, eating canned green beans is significantly better than eating no green beans at all. And since tomatoes are such an important part of the Mediterranean diet, you might even try canned whole plum tomatoes. The flavor is often much better than you get with so-called "fresh" tomatoes at the grocery store and their nutritional profile is still excellent. You can get varieties that are lower in salt, too. Eat more fruit as well. Start having fruit as your desert more and more often.

Of course, one way you can increase your consumption of fruits and vegetables is by juicing. Even though some of the juice proponents are way out of line with all the miracles that they're claiming, if it's easier for you to drink a glass of tomato or vegetable juice than it is to prepare a serving of vegetables, you're still getting the nutrients. But as I've said many times, it's better to eat the whole fruit than the juice. If, however, the only way I can get you to take in more fruits and vegetables is by juicing, and if your juicer does use the fiber and the pulp, that's a lot better than not getting the fruits or vegetables at all.

Of the fat you eat, try to go more with olive oil. Don't increase your overall fat intake, but of the fat you're currently eating, like from meat, butter, or margarine, take that fat and replace it with olive oil. Some of the research indicates that any monounsaturated fat works as well as olive oil does, so including canola oil would be fine as well. Instead of butter or margarine on your bread, sprinkle on a little bit of olive oil. Use it in salads and to sauté foods as well. You may need to experiment with the different flavors of olive oils. I recommend that you start with "extra light" olive oil; it's very mild in flavor and color and it appeals to a lot of American palates. Eventually, you might go with more of the traditional virgin or extra virgin olive oils. They have a stronger flavor and a darker color and are closer to traditional Mediterranean eating.

Next, start consuming more whole grain breads, cereals, pastas, and potatoes. If you're used to Wonder Bread right now, slowly work your way to whole grain. You don't have to accomplish this overnight, but eventually you want most of your grains to be whole. And remember you're looking for "100 percent whole wheat," not just "wheat" on a bread label. And let me say it one more time, just for the record, carbohydrates, close to the way they grow, are not fattening. They are the fundamental foundation upon which a good Mediterranean and American diet is based. Not white bread, not white flour. That's not how it grows.

The average Italian eats four times more bread than the average American. And yet you don't see near the obesity in Europe as you do in the US. Regardless of what the diet books that come and go may say, you want carbohydrates as the foundation of everything you eat every day. Yes, diabetics may have to watch their carb intake closer, but even then, whole grains are better than processed for them too. You don't have to be afraid of whole grain carbohydrates. And remember that fruits and vegetables are also carbohydrates.

Eat more salad. The Mediterraneans eat a lot of what they call "leaves."

> **DARK LEAFY GREENS OF ALL KINDS ARE LOADED WITH VITAMINS AND MANY OF THOSE PHYTOCHEMICALS THAT MAY PLAY A SIGNIFICANT ROLE IN DECREASING YOUR RISK OF THE BIG KILLERS.**

Eat more kinds of lettuce, spinach, turnip greens, mustard greens, Swiss chard, and purslane.

Remember the Mediterranean diet is not a vegetarian diet, they do eat chicken, fish, and meat, but at significantly lower frequencies and quantities than we do in the US. Low fat, lean meat can provide good nutrition, especially iron for women. You can add small amounts to pastas, rice, and beans, too. And you can also use it in making stews and hearty soups. But make it part of your recipes, not the centerpiece of the meal.

If you choose to drink alcohol, make it a glass of red wine and be sure to drink it with your meals. We're not exactly sure why that's important, but that does seem to be the consistent method of alcohol consumption. Rarely do you see alcohol consumed on an empty stomach in Mediterranean cultures.

And when it comes to dairy, the Mediterranean countries use less liquid milk than we do in the US. But they still use dairy in the form of yogurt and cheese. Remember that a traditional Italian pizza is not the same thing as you find here at Pizza Hut. In Italy it's not topped with cheese at all, but instead has tomato sauce, onions, peppers, herbs, and olive oil. The dough, not the toppings, is the centerpiece of a delicious pizza in Italy.

THE BIG PICTURE

Researchers now know that there isn't one particular component of the Mediterranean diet that makes it work. It's the combination of all the factors.

You can't just start using olive oil, for example, and expect benefit. The emphasis on the benefits on blood cholesterol levels from olive oil's monounsaturated fat content has probably been overstated. The lower cholesterol levels are more likely from the entire diet. The flavanoids of the red wine, the vitamin carotenoids, vitamin E, and vitamin C of the entire diet all have beneficial effects. The reduction of blood pressure is probably due, to a degree, to the fact that salt is primarily added in the kitchen, not in such high quantities from food processing as in the United States. It's the whole diet, and the whole lifestyle that seems to make the difference. Remember, it's not just eating like an Italian that will improve your health, it's living like them, too. That means you might need to spend a little more time in the kitchen making real foods instead of throwing something in the microwave.

It also means integrating physical activity in your lifestyle. But that doesn't necessarily mean going to a gym; it can mean working out in your garden, taking a nice relaxing walk in the evening, or walking down to the mail box two blocks instead of driving your car. The human body was designed to move and it appears that the people in the Mediterranean countries discovered that a long time ago. And they've got the health benefits as a result.

Remember in your journey of life that you're not an island; you're not in this alone. It's good for you to have social support, be it your church, some social group, or your family. Your wellness and longevity are positively affected when you interact in a healthy way with your fellow human beings. This can help in reducing stress and, with our hectic lifestyles today, stress is a major factor. And if there's any way you can swing it, a little break in the afternoon might also help.

Yes, this healthier approach to life can all take extra time, but you'll most likely get that time back in a longer, healthier life when you eat, and live, like an Italian.

A FINAL THOUGHT

Ten Bonus Years is all about prevention. By taking the steps you've learned here, you can dramatically increase your odds of living an additional decade of healthy life.

Isn't it true that you're more likely to accomplish something in life if you identify what your goal is? If you don't have a goal, your odds of accomplishing it by accident are relatively small. Think of those milestones in your life that you've accomplished; your education, your career, your family. They didn't just happen, you made them happen. Why can't that be true of longevity as well?

So, if you'd like to have an extra ten years of healthy life, why not make that your goal? This can dramatically change your attitude and your actions. Instead of looking at 70 as being old and at the end of life you begin to think of it as a time when you still have a lot of life left to live; you're not so ready to buy into the "old age" script. Instead, you realize that the best may still be ahead of you. If you practice what you've learned here scientists suggest you can add another healthy ten years to your life span. What would ten more healthy years be worth to you? I think it would be priceless.

ENERGIZE!
Your Next Meeting With
DAVID MEINZ

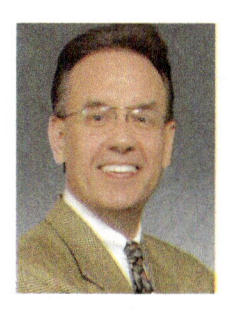

David Meinz will show your people how to improve their personal and professional productivity.

A CONTENT RICH, FUN, AND FUNNY PROGRAM!
- **The seven steps to increasing daily energy levels**
- **Surprising secrets about what you eat**
- **Living long and living well in the fast lane of life**

FOR BOOKING INFORMATION
Call us at 1-800-488-2857
www.DavidMeinz.com

And for David's most advanced program, be sure to visit
www.TheHealthyLifeSummit.com

CPSIA information can be obtained
at www.ICGtesting.com
Printed in the USA
FSOW03n0442190917
38638FS